DETOX
Yourself

DETOX
Yourself

JANE SCRIVNER

PIATKUS

© 1998 Jane Scrivner

First published in 1998 by
Judy Piatkus (Publishers) Ltd
5 Windmill Street
London W1P 1HF

Reprinted 1998 (four times)

The moral right of the author has been asserted
A catalogue record for this book is available from the British Library

ISBN 0-7499-1766-0

Designed by Paul Saunders

Typeset by Action Typesetting Limited, Gloucester
Printed and bound in Great Britain by Mackays of Chatham PLC

Contents

Introduction

Up until 1990 Penelope Lee and I worked together in the advertising industry. We put in long, hard hours and eventually decided that, if we were going to work at this level, we would prefer to do it for ourselves. We already had an active interest in complementary therapy, and this seemed the ideal way to combine a new start with an ongoing programme of 'improved quality of life'.

Complementary therapy is just as it says – a collection of therapies that can be used as preventative or curative measures to complement the more traditional Western medicines. It is this empowerment of the individual that makes complementary practice so attractive: if you don't feel well, or you have tried to find a solution to your condition and have been unsuccessful, complementary therapy will always be able to help. It may not provide a total cure every time, but it will provide the tools to make the situation better – massage for relaxation, reflexology for diagnostics, and so on.

Our bodies are the only things we have from day one right through until the end – we can't trade them in and we can't get new ones. We expect to get up every morning and work all day without a second thought. When things go wrong, we feel disappointed in our bodies and let down. But by making just small changes we can improve our lives and personal health dramatically, and at the same time greatly reduce the risk of ill health and things going wrong.

Due to popular demand from our clients we started to envisage a programme that would enable people to improve their lives and health in the comfort of their own homes. Over several years and after a lot of experimentation and revision we have devised what we feel is the ultimate plan to provide the required results. *Detox Yourself* is approachable, flexible, quite wonderfully indulgent and completely detoxifying! It is also quite simply the only natural way to get rid of that bane of so many women's lives, cellulite. Many of our clients have successfully completed the programme and the unanimous verdict is that they feel younger and healthier. There are very definite mental, physical, internal and external benefits, and they don't require anything except your own willingness to make the change.

The Detox Programme lasts thirty days and takes you through a carefully balanced eating and exercise regime, at the end of which you will feel cleansed, invigorated and like new. The changes don't need to be new or revolutionary – nearly every magazine you open contains 'Hints and Tips for a Better You' or features on detox tools such as dry skin brushing or fruit fasting, so it is likely that you have already heard of all the things included in this programme. Taken in isolation they can seem strange and confusing and possibly even bad for you, but put together in a formalised plan they can change your life!

The Detox Programme can also extend your life – by

the end of the thirty days you will have so much energy that we can guarantee at least a further hour each day. Now 365 hours is equal to fifteen days per year, so if you are interested in two weeks' extra holiday, then read on!

PART 1

Before you Begin

1

Why Detox?

'Detox starts with a change in your diet, building in relaxation, exercise and massage – it's about feeding the body, spirit and soul for life.'

A. Burnett, London

'The Detox Programme has given me renewed confidence in my appearance, high energy levels to cope with the pressures of my job and for once in my life a belief that I can change my diet successfully – thanks!'

D. Whittaker, London

WHY SHOULD I DETOX?

Two more hours per day, glowing skin, weight loss of several pounds, high energy levels, clear-headedness, higher thresholds for stress and tension, no cellulite, good body tone and a great feeling of being relaxed and totally in control of how you feel ... that's why you should detox.

Most people will agree that they don't feel totally 100 per cent. What are we doing to cause these feelings of lethargy and tiredness that we have become so used to? Generations have taken their bodies and health for granted and survived perfectly well, so why should we feel this way now?

Relatively recent developments mean we are more sophisticated in the way we live. Eating is an integral part of our lives, not just as a matter of survival but as a social activity too. Malnutrition in the West is rare. The food industry is so efficient that everything is available all year round, and we almost have too much choice. Our knowledge of food is much greater: most of us know what's good and what's bad. Stress levels are high, but no more so than for our parents. We are all aware of how important exercise is to maintaining fitness. So why do we get it so wrong? Why do we feel more like baked beans than spring beans?

Victims of our own success

We go to college or university, we have careers, we have families, we wear fashionable clothes, we 'do lunch', we entertain, we go on foreign holidays, we have wines and 'premium beers', we have long weekends away, we have deadlines ... what we don't have is a lot of time for ourselves. We don't sit and enjoy a nice quiet family lunch, we don't check our alcohol consumption, we don't cook or bake but buy convenience foods, we can't leave things until tomorrow, we skip meals, we grab a takeaway, we drive everywhere, we sit all day and we use tea and coffee to wake us up because we don't have time for an early night ... which is all fine – occasionally and in moderation. The 'modern' way of doing things, however, means we don't do things in moderation. We need to pack twice as much into every day, and we have devised short cuts to enable this to happen.

Preservatives, pre-packed foods, refined foods, fast foods, over-eating, under-eating, driving everywhere, bad posture, tight clothing, restrictive clothing ... the human body is wonderfully resourceful and will cope with quite a lot, but eventually things get out of control. If nothing is done, something has to give, and our bodies tell us with slow burn symptoms: dull skin, mouth ulcers, tiredness, weight loss, weight gain. If we choose to ignore the signs at this stage we are likely to go on to develop a more serious condition, but by acting on these warnings we can take full control and bring ourselves back to the peak of health.

WHAT DOES DETOX DO?

Detoxing or spring cleaning yourself is a preventative measure that will rid your body of the build-up of excess waste and toxins accumulated over the years.

- It will bring the control back into your life and the natural balance back into your body, thus getting you to your peak of health

- Everything in the programme is designed to fuel the body and teach it to use its own resources efficiently

- It provides the body with all the energy it requires to operate, and more to 'mend' any damage already caused

- It will rid your body of all the side-effects of our bad

habits, and will instil some ground rules that will mean you can indeed do twice as much in every day but without putting any unnecessary strain on your health

• It will cleanse your system

• It will enhance your circulation and improve your immune system

• It's the only way to get rid of your cellulite

HOW WILL IT DO THIS?

The Detox Programme feeds your body with the ultimate combination of foods. By closely following a recommended food list and exercise plan you can bring the body into total balance.

Many of the normal, everyday foods we eat can cause problems if we get too much or not enough. More extreme imbalances are well known, for instance lack of iron causing anaemia, too much alcohol causing addiction, and lack of vitamin C causing scurvy, but few of us are aware that very common foods can have a similar effect if not treated sensibly. Too many tomatoes can be too acidic and cause digestion problems. Because mushrooms are a fungus they can disrupt the delicate intestinal bacteria balance and weaken your ability to fight fungal infections. Orange juice can be hard work and congest your liver. And it is likely that any food you crave has become an allergen – your body has developed an intolerance to it.

During detox all 'extreme' foods are excluded, as are all

processed and refined foods. Everything is eaten in as natural and unprocessed a state as possible, and if it's not possible to do so in such a pure form the items in question are not included. No additives are allowed, and little if anything is taken away.

If it doesn't look like it was just picked, just dug up or just caught then don't eat it – it's not detox!

In addition to excluding all the 'bad' foods we include more of the 'good' foods that are often neglected or not recognised as being beneficial. There are many foods that can actively improve a condition or boost the general wellbeing of an individual that don't readily spring to mind as part of everyday eating:

- dried fruit
- raw vegetables
- potassium-rich foods
- garlic
- sprouted seeds and beans
- rice cakes
- hummus
- beetroot

as well as foods whose value is more commonly understood:

- fresh fruit

- fresh vegetables
- fish
- herbal teas
- pulses
- water

The road to total balance is not, however, followed purely through food and nutrition. With a view to increasing the efficiency of internal systems such as the liver, the kidneys, the circulation and the lymph glands, we will also look at:

- self-massage techniques
- dry skin brushing
- posture
- exercise
- breathing techniques
- magnesium bathing
- aromatherapy oils
- and many complementary ways to speed up the detox process

WILL IT BE DIFFICULT?

We are all creatures of habit. Introducing any change, no matter how small, needs concentration and effort. The Detox Programme should initially take thirty days. These thirty days in relation to the length of your life – that is, the length of your 'toxing' – is a very small amount of time.

The motivation of completely cleansing your internal systems and achieving all the benefits is great and you will start to feel the benefits by the end of the first seven days, if not sooner, but you should take the programme very seriously as an essential part of your own personal body maintenance plan. You owe this sort of programme to yourself. If you keep this positive frame of mind then the programme will only give benefits and will be easily enjoyed and adhered to. But if you decide that it will be an inconvenience and something that you have to 'shoe-horn' into twenty-eight days then perhaps you should reconsider and give the programme the priority it deserves – postpone it to a more convenient time or make more time now so that it can be accommodated more readily. The Detox Programme is one of the most positive steps you can take and should be treated and enjoyed that way – treat yourself!

How Long Does It Last?

How long is a piece of string? Detoxing should become a way of life!

The initial programme should last a minimum of thirty days, which allows sufficient time to 'spring clean' your body. If you try to do it in less time, the cleaning process is not completed and the results are not as satisfactory.

If you then undertake the total Detox Programme on a subsequent occasion you will begin to notice and 'feel' the signs that indicate you have detoxed completely. It is likely that this time around it will take less than the initial thirty days.

Ideally, as you begin to reach your thirty-day goal you will begin to decide which elements of the programme you will keep and which elements you will discontinue. Parts of the programme will stay with you forever, and parts will not be tried again.

It is likely that you will be about to embark on a very different way of eating, and elements of this will stay with you for the rest of your life. Foods that you enjoyed before the programme may not seem so enjoyable afterwards; this is generally due to their levels of toxins. Coffee is quite difficult to give up, but once you have spent thirty days without it, it is likely that the flavour will have become too strong or too processed for your newly revived palate. Similarly, foods that you might previously not have considered, such as rice cakes and fresh fish, will become a staple part of your eating plan.

There will also be times when you think that you may have overdone the high living and rich foods and feel like a one-week detox just to give your body a chance to recover some energy. Once you have completed the initial thirty-day programme it is entirely up to you to choose how to use the programme and tailor it to fit your lifestyle.

How Do You Feel?

Ultimately you will feel wonderful, as if you have much more energy at both ends of the day. When you wake up in the morning you may not wish to jump out of bed, but you won't feel lethargic or as if you need more sleep. You will be tired when you go to bed, but the feeling of exhaustion won't be there any more. You will sleep soundly and will wake less during the night. Your mind will feel fresh and the skin on both your face and body will feel smooth and toned. You will feel lean and much more aware of your body, the all-too-familiar 'fogginess' will have cleared and you will feel more vital.

You may experience some side-effects, but these really depend on how you lived prior to following the programme. If you were a heavy tea or coffee drinker you may experience one or two days of mild headaches as your body 'comes off' the caffeine. Similarly heavy sugar eaters, or heavy bread and pasta consumers, may experience a temporary energy loss as the body adjusts to the programme.

More general effects may be a small break-out of spots – not generally on the face. These show that the body is cleansing itself of all toxins: since the skin is the largest organ of the body it is the most obvious area for elimination and cleansing. A furry tongue is common in the early days but this will clear. Halitosis (bad breath) can also occur – again, only for a short time. All these symptoms indicate that the detox is working and can be helped with natural remedies, such as flushing the body with fluids and water, scraping the tongue every morning, and chewing parsley.

Other side-effects are generally due to misinterpreting the programme. For instance there may be occasions when you will feel tired, which probably means that you are not eating enough of the essential foods. These areas are covered fully in the relevant sections and more so in the troubleshooting checklist at the end of Chapter 4.

All the expected side-effects are positive indications that the programme is cleaning out your body and giving all your internal systems the valuable vitamins, minerals and nutrients they need to work at peak levels.

HOW DO I START?

Once you have decided to reward yourself with a new, revitalised, detoxed you, then read on. The following pages tell you everything you need to know and do prior to starting the programme, give you a step-by-step guide during the programme, and then offer plenty of ideas about how to maintain the programme once you have completed your initial thirty days.

Let's start with taking a look at how the body works and how waste and toxins affect us.

2

How the Body Functions

Before starting the Detox Programme it is worth knowing how the body operates and will respond to it. What causes the 'tox' to be there in the first place? What gets detoxed? And why does the body need our help – why doesn't it do the job itself?

First we need to look at the internal systems that will carry out your internal detox, and at what exactly makes up or causes the waste and toxins we are talking about. Only when you have understood these concepts and processes should you embark on the programme itself.

The human body is a highly sophisticated structure of organs and systems formulated to achieve balance and harmony. It uses foods and fluids for nourishment, repair and maintenance – what is known as metabolism. Our systems and organs process these foods, keep what they need and eliminate the waste – so, yes, the body does detox itself quite naturally. It is when we upset this balance, causing an overload of waste, that things can start to go wrong. The skin, liver, kidneys and lymph system are all critical to the smooth running of this process.

THE LIVER

Of the liver's several functions which are vital to health, two concern metabolism and detoxification. The liver takes the poisonous or toxic substances that enter our bodies via food or the environment and converts them to a form that the body can use, store safely or eliminate.

THE KIDNEYS

These organs are involved in many essential processes including filtering toxic wastes out of the blood and eliminating them from the body in urine. They are also responsible for maintaining the correct amount of fluid in the body and regulating the balance of potassium and sodium (vital for the correct flow of fluids in the systems).

THE LYMPH SYSTEM

This system acts as a waste disposal facility for the body. Lymph, a liquid produced by lymph glands in various parts of the body, absorbs dead cells, excess fluids and other waste products from foods and takes them to the lymph nodes. Here the waste is filtered and eventually fed into the blood and on to one of the eliminatory organs – skin, liver or kidneys – to be passed out via perspiration, faeces or urine.

THE SKIN

This is the largest organ in the body and serves many vital functions.

A mirror to our health

The skin can be a useful indicator of what is happening within our bodies. 'Looking a bit pale', 'Looking well', 'Glowing', and 'In the pink' are all everyday phrases used to describe our health through looking at our skin.

If the skin mirrors what is happening internally, it is said that the chin area reflects exactly what is happening in the stomach and gut – in other words it reflects your diet and what you are eating. We have all had a break-out of nasty spots on our chins at some time or another, and if you think back it will generally relate to an unhealthy period of eating or drinking!

If we are under stress, our skin looks tired and pale. If we are ill, the skin loses colour. If we are severely ill, jaundice (yellowing of the skin), lesions or weeping wounds are just some extreme examples of what can occur.

Excretion

As an organ of elimination the skin is a mere beginner in relation to the liver and kidneys, but it still excretes large quantities of waste products: water, salts, uric acid, ammonia and urea. The skin is like a huge sieve or colander – the goodness stays in and the waste passes out. If the liver and kidneys are overworked or not working efficiently the result may be skin complaints such as eczema, due to the skin having to deal with more waste than normal.

Protection

The skin protects our bodies in many ways. It forms a physical barrier against 'foreign' substances. It produces an acidic secretion which kills off harmful micro-organisms. It is semi-permeable and regulates what can enter and exit the body. And it prevents excess water loss so as to avoid dehydration.

Body temperature

Our skin regulates our body temperature. If we get hot through exercise or because we are in a hot environment our bodies produce sweat, and this cools the skin and body as it evaporates from the surface of the skin. If we get cold, our blood vessels dilate and reduce the flow of blood to the top layers of the skin, thus reducing the loss of heat.

Warning signals

Our skin is our early warning system against danger. If we touch something too hot or too cold, the skin sends messages to the brain to withdraw or take appropriate action.

THE BODY IN BALANCE

Our long-term health relies on keeping ourselves and our bodies in balance, so that any undue stress or strain that the body experiences can be dealt with efficiently and the body can return to normal after a short period of recovery. If any one of the organs or systems described above is not fully functional, things begin to slow down and can eventually result in an overload of waste and toxins.

A body that is out of balance will need considerably longer to recover, as more strain is being put on the systems to process the excess waste and toxins – feelings of being 'under par' and tired become more frequent. However, if the body is fully fit and healthy the amount of waste matter to be dealt with is at normal levels and this processing is under control, so we feel well and have plenty of energy.

The detox process is designed to keep all these eliminatory organs in tip-top tone and condition – in short, in balance.

How do we get out of balance?

There are many ways to throw this careful harmony off course, and they all contribute to overloading the eliminatory organs and systems with waste and toxins or slowing them down, both of which can result in their malfunction.

Some forms of waste and toxins occur naturally in the body:

- Through metabolism, every day the body processes and eliminates billions of worn out and dead cells quite normally

- The body processes all excess fluid that is no longer required

- Following illness or injury, the body eliminates dead or scar tissue

None of these waste products should be interfered with, as they are crucial to a normal healthy body. However, there are several areas where we can consciously decrease the introduction of waste into our bodies:

- Being unfit can slow down your metabolic rate and so decrease the detox activity within your body

- Being ill will mean that the body functions are disturbed and concentrating on recovery; again this will slow down the internal detox process

- Eating badly or eating only fast foods means the body doesn't get all the necessary nutrients

- Being under stress puts the body into fight-or-flight mode (see p.20)

There are also many waste products, toxins and situations that we can and should avoid:

- Cigarettes, alcohol, caffeine and drugs are all products that the body cannot absorb and use and so they add to the mounting levels of waste

- A diet too high in fats and sugars will add to the waste

- The environment adds to the waste – pollution, exhaust fumes and pesticides are just some of the culprits

- Over the past century we have developed the food manufacturing industry in such a way that the numbers and quantities of additives and preservatives have increased phenomenally in our now more sophisticated, more complicated diet

- We also refine the goodness out of many of the original basic nutritional foodstuffs and eat refined wheat, refined flour, refined sugar and so on

Most of us can say that some or all of these are currently a regular part of our diet and lifestyle. This means that we now consume many types of food that the body cannot assimilate and many chemicals that, if not eliminated, will act as toxins in the body. This situation increases the number of food types that the body leaves partially or totally undigested, and so increases the levels of waste that the body has to deal with to remain healthy and in balance.

All this excess waste needs to be eliminated, but if there is too much for the body to deal with a build-up will result. In high concentrations these waste materials become toxic and can 'poison' the body. In a healthy, fit person the body can assimilate and eliminate all wastes and toxins. In a tired, unhealthy or ill body, the build-up of this waste will start to affect the efficiency of the organs and lead to sluggishness, fatigue and eventually illness. It is this build-up that the Detox Programme will initially decrease and eventually, through new eating habits, erase completely so that our bodies are only being given foods that they can use or eliminate naturally.

STRESS AS A CONTRIBUTING FACTOR

Stress changes the body's normal state, but we need a degree of stress in order to be alert and active to prepare and deal with outside stimuli. Stress causes a natural 'fight-or-flight' reaction in our bodies – we become immediately responsive by either running away or fighting back, and this protects us from danger or difficult situations.

The body reacts to stress by sending a hormone called adrenaline to the legs (to enable us to run away) or to the shoulders and upper torso muscles (to enable us to physically fight the enemy). This was good for our cave man ancestors, whose problems were not those of deadlines or traffic jams but those of hunting food or being eaten themselves! They used up all this adrenaline quickly, but when we are put under pressure today we stay in a prolonged state of alertness which, if it continues without rest, will have a damaging effect on our bodies.

At this time of stress the body needs all its resources and so all the other bodily systems temporarily slow down or cease. Blood, for instance, moves away from the digestive system to the muscles in order to prepare for physical action, the bowels empty, the heart rate increases, blood pressure increases, sweating occurs, the pupils dilate, the mouth becomes dry as food is not required – in short, the body has turned away from the essential processes of digestion and absorption of foods and nutrients for repair and maintenance in favour of self-defence.

Remaining in a prolonged state of stress will result in undigested food, the secreting of toxins by the body, and slow and inefficient processing of the waste products in the body. All this causes excess and overload which, if not dealt with quickly, will simply build up each time the body is subjected to further stress.

Part of the Detox Programme involves getting rid of, or

at least managing, some of the stress in our lives in order to minimise the unnecessary disturbance of our bodies.

What physically happens when there is a build-up or overload of waste, toxins and stress?

The human body is very sophisticated and will still function well under some extremely adverse conditions. The build-up of stress, waste and toxins happens very gradually and the body will adapt to these new conditions. But each time it is required to adapt, some of the efficiency is lost. Eventually we start to get warning signs that it is time to implement some changes ourselves before irreversible damage is caused.

The overload of toxins in the system will generally result in a feeling of fatigue, both physically and mentally. This is caused by each of the eliminatory organs/systems having its own problems as a build-up of waste occurs – each organ or system reacts differently. Below are some of the more obvious effects that are pertinent to the Detox Programme.

Extended periods of stress will cause extended periods of poor nutrition, bad absorption, increased blood pressure and heart rate and inefficient functioning of the bodily systems. Nutrition, repair and maintenance soon become replaced with basic survival, and the internal eliminatory organs become sluggish in their processing of undigested foods and waste. As the body deals with stress we feel exhausted and mentally drained.

The liver takes potentially damaging substances that we have introduced into our daily routines, such as alcohol, drugs, poisons and caffeine, and breaks them down into forms that can be eliminated via the faeces and urine. The liver also takes toxic substances produced by the body and removes them by elimination to prevent self-poisoning. If the liver becomes overworked and inefficient illnesses such as jaundice and gallstones can occur.

If the blood contains too many toxins and waste products the kidneys will have to work hard, and if we don't take optimum care of these organs this may lead to their sluggish or inefficient functioning. If any of these functions fail, serious illness will result. In the same way, if any of these functions cause the kidneys to be overworked the result can be tiredness and lethargy.

Poor lymph drainage due to excess waste results in a build-up of fluid containing waste products. As we know, this waste can become toxic and stagnant and eventually will induce feelings of bloating and fatigue. In addition, tissue can be damaged due to the excess fluid.

How do we prevent this build-up or overload of waste and toxins?

It is likely, if you are reading this book, that you have already got a certain build-up of toxins. You may not be aware of any actual feelings of illness, but you may have some side-effects of a gradual build-up: tiredness, lethargy, irritable bowel, mouth ulcers, spots and blemishes, dull complexion, low energy levels, bloated feelings, fluid retention, muscle fatigue, heavy periods or headaches.

Avoiding the causes of waste is not always easy, but by following a carefully planned eating programme and being aware of your surroundings you can greatly reduce them. A formalised detoxification programme will not only provide the body with unprocessed, pure foods but also concentrate on specific foods that will actively create the ideal environment for your body to regain its natural balance. Such a programme will also cover all complementary activities that enhance the food aspects: stress reduction and management, exfoliation, breathing, massage, exercise and so on. Once you have eliminated all toxins from your body, you will be in a much better position to maintain this status and keep the balance.

Now that you have a basic understanding of how the body functions, of what wastes and toxins are, how they affect our bodies and what we can do to avoid them, you are ready to start!

3

Preparing for Detox

BEFORE COMMENCING THE PROGRAMME

There are few reasons why you should not start the Detox Programme, but these reasons are very important indeed and should always be considered. You should not start the programme if any of the following applies to you at the time of your detox:

- You are pregnant

- You are breastfeeding

- You are undergoing medical treatment for any illness or condition

- You are recovering from a serious illness

- You are taking any prescribed or non-prescribed drugs

- You have any doubts about your own medical health

Always consult your doctor if you are in any doubt as to whether this programme is suitable for you.

How to Plan the Thirty Days

When you have decided that you want to detox, the first thing to work out is how much of a change from your normal way of eating it is going to be. Doing a short self-assessment will enable you to see if there are some extra things that you might want to start a few weeks in advance of the programme itself. Doing so may make the programme less of a shock to the system and therefore ultimately easier and more enjoyable. If you complete the following questions you can work out the best way to start your own detox. Circle or tick the alternative that best describes your current situation.

Self-assessment

How do you rate your current diet?
(Score 3) Very healthy
(Score 2) Fairly healthy
(Score 1) Bad

How are your energy levels?
(Score 3) Good
(Score 2) OK
(Score 1) Low

Which best describes your activity levels?
(Score 3) Regular exercise and/or an active job or life
(Score 2) Some exercise but a sedentary job
(Score 1) No exercise and a sedentary job

How much water do you drink per day?
(Score 3) 3 pints/(1.7 litres)
(Score 2) 3–4 glasses
(Score 1) Fewer than 3 glasses

How much coffee, tea or canned drinks (cola etc.) do you drink per day?
(Score 3) Few/none
(Score 2) About 3
(Score 1) About 6 or more

How much alcohol do you drink per week? (one unit equals a medium glass of wine, a pint of beer or lager, or one measure of spirits)
(Score 3) 4–6 units
(Score 2) 8–12 units
(Score 1) 15 units or more

How much fresh fruit or vegetables do you eat every day?
(Score 3) 3–4 portions
(Score 2) 1–2 portions
(Score 1) 1/none

Now add your scores together and interpret them as follows:

Scores above 14

If you have scored above 14 on the self-assessment you should be able to start the Detox Programme on Day 1 as described, without any further preparation.

Scores below 14

If you have scored below 14 on the self-assessment you should consider making some changes before you embark on Day 1. In the month before detox consider changing your daily life along these lines:

- Start doing some mild exercise, such as a walk at lunchtime or running up and down the stairs five times before bed – anything that will increase your pulse rate for twenty minutes each day

- Make sure you drink at least 2 pints (1 litre) of water a day

- Reduce your alcohol intake by half

- Reduce your intake of coffee, tea and fizzy drinks by half

- Make sure you eat at least three portions of fruit and three portions of vegetables each day. A portion of fruit is an apple or a pear etc., and a portion of vegetables is one large serving spoon or more.

WHEN TO START

Ideally you need to allocate your thirty days well in advance. The early part of the year is often a good time – once you have recovered after Christmas the next few months are a time for taking stock, making life decisions and saving money! Depending on when Easter falls, February or March are good candidates. There are plenty of fruit and vegetables around and the spring and summer social occasions have not yet started – weekends away, barbecues, summer children's parties and so on.

Try to find a start time when you have relatively few social commitments. Beginning the programme on the weekend of your best friend's wedding is likely to push your self-control to its limits, and turning up with a Tupperware container full of rice and veggies may prove a subject for discussion but will ultimately ruin the day!

There is no need to take time off work. But again, if you know that you have a run of meetings or conferences coming up and will be subject to caterers' food this is a time to avoid.

If your child's birthday party is on the horizon or you are hosting the local coffee morning, think twice about starting the programme. This is not because the programme is hard to keep to, but it is a departure from your normal lifestyle and you will make extra work if you spend most of the time avoiding or adapting to fit these occasions.

The best day to start is a Sunday. Plan to have a relatively quiet time at work for the next week or so, don't make any social arrangements in the first week, and thereafter try to keep to close friends and entertaining at home – you can easily entertain friends without them ever knowing they are 'on the detox' for the evening. (Chapter 5 is full of useful recipes for such occasions.) Once you have got into the swing of the programme you will be able to plan the remaining days to suit yourself. By the end of the first week you will be much more aware of what you should be eating, and you will have found a routine for the other activities.

MENTAL PREPARATION

The time when you detox is a time you should enjoy – you deserve to find time for yourself, and you should look upon the Detox Programme as a treat for yourself and your body. Don't think that there are lots of things that you can't have, but that there are lots of things you can. There will be new foods for you to try, lots of ways that you can pamper your body, lots of ways to reduce or manage stress, tools to get rid of cellulite and a chance to feel much healthier and much more vital.

So think of the Detox Programme as your own personal month at a health farm – you will be creating your own 'Detox Oasis'. Enjoy each day of the programme. Don't always think about how long you have to go, but think about how much you have already done and how good you feel. When you tell people what you are doing they will be very interested. Don't tell them how different it is from normal and how time-consuming it is to get everything done, but tell them how many positive changes you have made and how you are doing much more every day due to your increased energy levels. Adopting a positive state of mind from the start will make the programme much more satisfying – 'getting through' the programme will make it feel like a struggle and you are more likely to give up or leave the programme incomplete.

PHYSICAL PREPARATION

Although you should be able to follow the programme quite normally without having to buy or use any special equipment, there are some things that you need to gather or source. Many of these you will already have or will know where to get hold of, but you should do this in plenty of time. Having them ready when you start makes the programme go smoothly; a little preparation is in any case never a bad thing and certainly a good habit to get into.

Checklist of essentials

- **Airtight food or Tupperware containers**

  A variety of sizes is useful as you can store large amounts (rice etc.) or carry small snacks for when you are on the move

- **Steamer – metal or bamboo**

  The type you put over or in a pan of hot water to steam vegetables or fish

- **Skin brush – natural bristles**

  Bristles should be firm but not too stiff, otherwise they may irritate the flesh

- **Exfoliating creams or salt**

  Use up any odds and ends of creams to save money. If they are not exfoliants, add a teaspoon of salt or sand and this will do the job

- **Loofah or flannel mitt**

  Towelling or natural fibre

- **Moisturising creams**

  Anything you have at home – take the opportunity to use up all the old bottles of moisturiser that have been hanging around and you haven't thrown away yet

- **Massage creams or oils**

  Any natural oils are suitable. If you have massage oils these are fine but sunflower, olive or grapeseed oils from the supermarket or your kitchen cupboards are all great. They are better than cosmetic creams because, being natural products, they will be completely absorbed into the flesh

- **Somewhere to exercise**

  Gym, bedroom, stairs, lounge etc.

- **Bath or shower**

  Access to both a bath and a shower is ideal, but one or the other is fine

Checklist of optionals/luxuries

- **Sauna or steam room**

  See if there is one in your local leisure centre. It will be cheaper than a health club and using it can be combined with a swim

- **Juicer**

  This is an absolute luxury, but what better time to try than during the detox?

- **Weekend or day trip to the sea or countryside**

  Breathing fresh air is one of the best things for the Detox Programme – time away is always beneficial

- **Organic foods**

  There are many suppliers of organic fruit, veg and fish prepared to supply nationally. Using organic foods will guarantee that all pesticides are eliminated before you even start. Organic foods are not essential – the fact that you are going to be eating fresh foods over the next month is probably enough of a change, but if fruit and vegetables already form the basis of your diet then try organics and see if you notice a difference

The following topics will be discussed at length in Chapter 9, but it may be worth sourcing them before you start. There is a list of contact numbers on page 192 which should help you to find practitioners in your area.

- **Massage, aromatherapy**   You may be able to find these locally or, even better, some practitioners will do home visits

- **Colonic irrigation**   Your local health centre should be able to help you locate local practitioners

- **Reflexology**   Again, your local health centre or even health food shop may be able to give you names of local practitioners

There are some more unusual items – on top of your meals – that you will be required to eat or drink every day, and these should be bought in advance as you are unlikely to have them in stock. They are listed here merely for shopping purposes, and will be fully explained in Chapter 4. Some may sound a bit odd, but all will be revealed later!

Essential shopping

- **Vegetable juice – carrot or beetroot**

  Bottled juice is usually available from health food shops. Start with one bottle. Alternatively, if you have a juicer buy fresh vegetables and juice your own

- **Olive oil**

  Try to buy extra virgin, cold pressed or first pressed oils as these are purer and contain the highest nutrients. They are available in all supermarkets. One or two pints (1 litre) will do to start

- **Fresh garlic and odourless garlic pills**

  From greengrocers, health food shops and some supermarkets. To start, buy enough pills to take one a day, or a large bulb so that you can eat one clove a day

- **Honey**

  Buy one pot, preferably from someone who stocks or produces good-quality, home-made honey. The less refined the honey the better, so look for cold-pressed

- **Fresh lemons**

  From greengrocers or supermarkets. Buy three to start

- **Sprouted beans**

  From health food shops, or buy a sprouter and do your own. You can also sprout your own beans on absorbent paper: simply dampen the paper, sprinkle the seeds over it and leave in a light, sunny place. Make sure the paper doesn't dry and the beans will sprout in a few days. Mung beans, chick peas and alfalfa are all good. If you cannot find these, replace them with a daily supplement of alfalfa pills

- **A hot spice of your choosing**

  Choose one or several spices, chilli, cayenne, lemon grass, ginger – raw is best, but powder will do

- **Water**

  Filtered or bottled. Still is preferable to fizzy, which can be saved for evenings out. You will need enough for 3 pints a day (1.7 litres) for the first three days. Use tap water in emergencies only – when there is no other kind available

You can gather these items together in preparation for Day 1, but the bulk of the foodstuffs should be bought as and when you would normally do your shopping. The fresher the foods, the more nutrients you will get. Fresh, crisp vegetables will leave you feeling fresh and crisp yourself; old, limp vegetables ... need I say more?

WHAT IT COSTS

If you don't have some or all of the 'essential items', try to borrow them from friends to keep costs down. But if you do buy, these won't be wasted purchases as you will probably continue to use them long after the programme is over. A steamer, plastic containers and skin brushes or flannels should together cost less than a good facial – which you will not need as the detox will leave your skin radiant and pure.

The essential food extras such as vegetable juice and olive oil may mean spending up front, but you will recoup the money during the programme as your fresh foods will cost less than the processed foods that you would normally buy.

PART 2

Time to Detox

4

The Detox Programme

'The diet looked pretty daunting, but I found it quite easy to follow and actually enjoyed it. As well as following the programme, I had to use a body brush, shower in cold water every morning, have massages and take exercise. The results were great. I lost half a stone in the first three weeks and definitely noticed a reduction in my cellulite. It's hard work, but I would do it again – it has been an education.'

Jane, London

Make sure you read this section several times. There will always be things on the lists that you will forget or combinations that you do not realise, and reading several times before and during the programme will ensure that you don't miss any of these. There is a checklist at the end of this chapter for you to use every day.

The Detox Programme is a 'total body experience'. The approach is holistic and works on every part of the body – internal and external.

- There are foods that work on specific areas of the body and as such should be included in the programme every day – do not miss these out

- There are body care routines that should be followed every day – again, do not miss these out

FOODS ON THE DETOX PROGRAMME

The Detox Programme is very specific: if the foods are not listed in the next few pages, they are not included in the programme. You do not need to be a whizz in the kitchen, but do try to be as varied as possible in your food choices as this will make the programme more interesting. In the same way that you probably follow a routine in your meals at the moment – for instance, toast and coffee for breakfast, sandwiches for lunch and a pasta dish for supper – it is completely normal to fall into a routine of having a similar thing each lunchtime and so on whilst you are on the programme – just try to make the ingredients slightly different each day. The following sections will take you through:

- Foods you must have every day and why

- Everything you can eat for the full thirty days, by category

- Foods you think would be included but are most definitely not, and why

When you start the Detox Programme, from Day 1 to Day 30 you must:

- Drink a cup of hot water and lemon juice first thing every morning

- During the day drink 3 pints (1.7 litres) of water
- Take two liver tonics as described on p.43
- Take two kidney tonics as described on p.43
- Take kelp supplements every day
- Take multivitamin supplements every day for the first fifteen days
- Eat at least three meals every day from the food lists
- Have at least one portion of rice every day – preferably short grain brown rice
- Have at least three portions of vegetables – one should be raw
- Have at least three portions of raw or dried fruit
- Have at least three portions of salad
- Have at least one portion of non-dairy yoghurt, cheese or milk every day. (Non-dairy means goat's or sheep's products, rice products (i.e. rice milk) or soya products (i.e. soya milk)
- Have two portions every day of either pulses, nuts, herbs, olive or any seed oil, or fish

Why you need these foods and this regime

Hot lemon water The biggest organ of detox is the liver, and starting the day with a squeeze of fresh lemon juice in a cup of hot water will not only refresh and revitalise you but will also clean your palate and 'jump start' your liver. The lemon is also alkaline, which will help to balance the pH in your system during detox. People in many Eastern cultures scrape the surface of their tongue first thing in the morning in the belief that doing so greatly reduces the amount of infections and germs that they carry. You may want to try this, but if not swill the first mouthful of lemon water and spit it out before drinking the rest as normal. Cider vinegar can be substituted, but may be a little sharp for most palates.

Water Around 80 per cent of our bodies consists of water and we need to keep that level stable. In hot weather or during exercise you should increase this amount to cover the deficit. Water replenishes, cleanses, rejuvenates and restores, and is probably the most important single item in the Detox Programme. At first the essential 3 pints (1.7 litres) may feel too much, and you will spend a lot of time going to the bathroom! After a few days your body will become used to the amount and will start to ask for more by making you thirsty. You must be sure to spread this intake of water over the whole day – drinking it all in one go will put pressure on your internal organs and is not healthy. Reduce the amount you drink leading up to bedtime so that you won't have to get up during the night.

'At first it was difficult to get used to eating very different types of food and I was also surprised how long it took me to get used to no caffeine – I had a mild headache for nearly five days, which indicated just how much I used to drink without thinking about it. It was all worth it as I have never felt livelier, brighter or more energised.'

Joyce, London

Liver tonics The liver should be treated with tender loving care over the thirty-day programme. There are many ways to do this but you may find that some are more acceptable than others for your own personal tastes. Each of the foods listed below will cleanse the liver and act as a tonic for it. If you want to include all of them in your programme that's fine, but you must take at least two each day – vary them from day to day if you wish.

- Eat a medium bunch of black grapes

- Eat a fresh garlic clove (in foods, not on its own), or take an odourless garlic tablet – a high-dose tablet is best

- Drink a medium glass of pure carrot and beetroot juice. You can juice this yourself or buy fresh juices from health food shops

- Drink two cups of fennel or dandelion tea

Kidney tonics The other major detox organs are the kidneys. Daily eating or drinking of specific foods that will boost the kidneys will help the overall programme. Again, you may vary your choice but you must have two per day:

- Slowly sip a teaspoon of fresh honey dissolved in a cup of hot water

- Drink a medium glass of freshly squeezed cranberry juice (you may wish to add some honey to sweeten it) or take a cranberry tablet supplement. Fresh cranberries are generally only available in the winter, although frozen berries are available all year round

- Eat half a medium melon, but do not combine it with any other foods for up to half an hour before or afterwards as it may cause indigestion

'I have so much more energy. For the first time in years I feel as if my body is firing on all cylinders.'

P. Thomas, London

Kelp supplements Kelp, a kind of seaweed, provides the body with good quantities of iodine, which keeps the metabolic rate balanced. When we make any changes in our eating habits we often affect our metabolic rate, and if we do not eat enough or exercise enough it will begin to slow down. Iodine will keep the metabolism steady and effective for detox.

Multivitamin supplements Vitamin supplements will ensure that any problems or shortfalls in the early stages of the programme will not leave the body short of essential nutrients. But after fifteen days you can stop as by this stage your body will be getting all essential nutrients from the programme.

Three meals a day Eating three meals a day is becoming less and less common: we tend to skip breakfast, have lunch on the hoof and grab supper late at night. But during the programme you must eat three meals every day.

Ideally, breakfast should be before 9 a.m., lunch before 2 p.m. and the evening meal before 7 p.m. This allows sufficient time for your body to process the food before the next meal, and to process all the foods eaten that day before the start of the following day. (In a healthy body foods should normally take less than twenty-four hours to go from eating to defecation, but most people take more than twice that time to process what they eat.)

Brown rice Rice is one of the most absorbent carbohydrates we can have in our diet. It also seems not to give rise to the allergic reactions and intolerances that many wheat-based carbohydrates cause. Being absorbent, it can act as a 'plunger' for our intestines. Imagine your household pipes after twenty years of use – it is likely that they have either corroded or you have had to call in a plumber to sort out minor and major blockages. As rice travels through the gut it collects all the silt and waste on the way and then flushes it out. And when you are detoxing, it means that each time waste is removed in this way it is not replaced – each time you eat absorbent rice it will break away a little more of the accumulated waste until the gut is completely cleansed.

Short grain brown rice is the most absorbent kind and should be used throughout the programme. If there are occasions, for instance when eating out, when short grain is not available, then long grain brown or wild rice are the next best options. White rice should be eaten only in absolute desperation! NB: this is the only concession on the programme – substitutes should not be used for any other foods. Remember: if it's not on the list, you must not eat it.

Other foods on the detox list The remaining ingredients in all your meals will consist entirely of fruit, vegetables, salads, herbs, fish, nuts, pulses, seeds and goat's or sheep's cheeses/yoghurts etc., or their vegan equivalent. In order to get a healthy spread of necessary nutrients you must have some of each of these foods every day. If you miss out on a food category you may begin to feel lethargic, as something essential to your daily requirements will be missing. You don't need to have everything for every meal but a sensible combination could be fruit for breakfast, fish salad for lunch, roast vegetables and rice for supper, nuts for a mid-morning snack, and goats' cheese and rice cakes for dessert. Try to vary this as much as possible, but make sure you eat it all. It is important to include raw foods as well as lightly cooked foods, for raw foods provide bulk and fibre that will increase the body's ability to detox.

'I discovered the joy of early mornings – I woke at least an hour earlier, refreshed and ready to go!'

F. Wheatley, Devon

THE FOOD LISTS

Fruit and vegetables: the specifics

Both fruit and vegetables are high in nutrients as they contain large amounts of essential vitamins, amino acids and minerals. They have high fibre and high potassium, but contain very little waste and very few calories. Fruit and vegetables consist nearly entirely of goodness. You should aim to eat fresh fruit and vegetables as fresh as possible. The longer you store them the more nutrients are lost, and certainly as soon as you begin to process them yourself the goodness will disappear quickly. Raw food equates to raw energy; raw food cleans the gut more efficiently; and raw food contains high levels of dietary fibre. So you should attempt to eat as much of your fruit and vegetable quota in its raw state. If this is impossible then make sure that a high percentage is raw, for instance salad with lightly steamed vegetables, or grated raw carrot and beetroot over a bowl of grilled vegetables. Fruit can be eaten fresh or dried.

The fruit list

Apples
Apricots
Bilberries
Blackberries
Blackcurrants
Blueberries
Cherries
Cranberries
Currants (dried and fresh)
Damsons
Dates
Figs
Gooseberries

Grapefruit
Grapes
Greengages
Guavas
Kiwi fruit
Lemons
Limes
Loganberries
Lychees
Mangoes
Melons
Mulberries
Nectarines
Passion fruit

Paw-paw
Peaches
Pears
Pineapple
Plums
Pomegranates
Prunes
Quinces
Raisins
Raspberries
Redcurrants
Rhubarb
Strawberries
Sultanas

The vegetable list

Artichokes, globe
and Jerusalem
Asparagus
Aubergines (eggplant)
Beans, French,
runner, broad,
butter, haricot,
mung and
red kidney
Bean sprouts
Beetroot
Broccoli
Brussels sprouts
Cabbage, red, savoy,
spring, white and
winter
Carrots

Cauliflower
Celeriac
Celery
Chicory
Chinese leaf
Courgettes (zucchini)
Cucumber
Fennel
Kohlrabi
Leeks
Lettuce, all types
Marrow
Okra (ladies'
fingers)
Onions
Parsnips
Peas, all types

Peppers (bell
peppers, capsicums)
Plantain
Potatoes
Pumpkin
Radishes
Spring greens
Spring onions
(scallions)
Swede
Sweetcorn (corn on
the cob, maize)
Sweet potatoes
Squashes
Turnips
Watercress
Yams

Nuts: the specifics

Although high in calories, nuts are also extremely high in
nutrients and an excellent source of essential unsaturated
fatty acids, and are a rich source of potassium and fibre.
The following nuts should be eaten raw, unsalted and
fresh.

The nut list

Almonds
Brazils
Cashews
Chestnuts

Hazelnuts
Macadamia nuts
Pecans

Pine nuts
Pistachio nuts
Walnuts

Pulses, seeds, herbs and spices: the specifics

Pulses and seeds are high in nutrients and once they are freshly sprouted the nutrient content becomes even higher. When a seed has sprouted it is easier to digest, being partially digested already. Seeds and sprouts add flavour and colour to our foods, but their vitamin and nutrient content is of ultimate importance. Herbs should ideally be fresh so that you get the benefit of all their nutrients. Dried herbs will supply flavour but little else.

The pulse, seed, herb and spice list

Alfalfa	Fennel	Rosemary
Basil	Ginger, fresh	Sage
Cardamom pods	and powdered	Sesame seeds
Cayenne pepper	Lemon grass	Sunflower seeds
Chick peas	Marjoram	Tarragon
Chillies	Parsley	Thyme
Coriander, fresh	Pepper, fresh	
and powdered	ground	
Dill	Pumpkin seeds	

Non-dairy: the specifics

Non-dairy is an odd term but it best describes the fermentation process, which is different from that used in cow's milk production. The process means that goat's and sheep's products are much easier to digest and can also aid digestive disorders and actually stimulate digestion. Many people who have developed an allergy to cow's milk products will find they have no reaction from either sheep's or goat's milk products.

The non-dairy list

Goat's cheese	Sheep's milk	Soya milk
Sheep's cheese	Goat's yoghurt	Rice milk
Goat's milk	Sheep's yoghurt	

Fish: the specifics

All fish contain essential proteins, but oily fish such as herrings, mackerel and salmon has the added benefit of the oils. Wherever possible you should eat fresh fish. If fresh is not available or you are using canned fish for convenience, the best varieties are those canned in olive or vegetable oil. Some fish is canned in spring water, but check that no salt has been added. If it has, then make sure the fish is drained completely and rinsed before eating. Fish in brine is too salty and should not be used on the detox. Smoked fish is acceptable but should be naturally smoked and not dyed or coloured. Frozen can be used for convenience, but it will have lost some nutrients. Fresh is always best and will contain the most nutrients.

The fish list

Cod	Mackerel	Sardines
Crab	Monkfish	Scampi
Haddock	Pilchards	Shrimps
Halibut	Plaice	Skate
Herring	Prawns	Trout
Lemon sole	Salmon	Tuna
Lobster		

Drinks: the specifics

During the programme you are required to drink 3 pints (1.7 litres) of water per day. If the water becomes a little repetitive, you can use some natural flavourings to make it more interesting. Try honey, or lemon. Juices are not counted as water but can be drunk in addition to the required amounts. If you are buying ready-squeezed juices, try to get pure juice in preference to juice made up in water from fruit pulp – it will say on the carton or bottle. If you find the juice too strong, dilute to taste with water – it makes the juice go further and increases your water intake all at once.

The drinks list

Herbal teas, any
Honey in water
Lemon juice in
 water

Juices, freshly
squeezed,
pure and
unsweetened,
apple or grape or
any juiced vegetable

Water, hot, cold,
fizzy and spring,
with tap water
for emergencies
only

Miscellaneous foods: the specifics

These are the items that are hard to categorise. They are, however, just as essential to the programme as the foods listed earlier, as they too add nutrients, variety and flavour. Try to include as many of these as possible. Tahini can be bought from most health food stores. You can choose between 'light' tahini, sesame seeds that are hulled before being ground, or 'dark' tahini, which simply means that the hulls have been left on. Make sure that your tahini is unsalted – most are, but it is worth checking on the ingredients.

The miscellaneous list

Balsamic vinegar	Olive oil	Seaweed
Cider vinegar	Olives, green	Sesame oil
Grapeseed oil	or black	Tahini
Miso	Quorn	Tofu
Mustard, grain	Rice cakes,	Walnut oil
not powder	unsalted	

Common foods you cannot have

Oranges are excluded from the programme because they are the most acidic of all fruit. Their close relatives, however (tangerines, satsumas etc.), are less acidic and can be included on the Detox Programme. Acidity is harmful to the liver and foods containing large amounts of acids should be avoided. Contrary to what you might think, grapefruits, limes and lemons are all alkaline producing foods, and so are included in the programme.

Avocados	*Too much starch and fat*
Bananas	*Too much starch and fat*
Bread	*Gluten in the wheat flour can be difficult to digest*
Caffeine	*Chemical stimulant*
Chocolate	*Too much sugar and fat*
Cow's milk/cheese, etc.	*Lactose (milk sugar) can be difficult to digest*
Lentils	*Too much gas*
Mushrooms	*Too much fungus*
Oranges	*Too acidic*

Peanuts	*Too much fat and starch*
Salt	*Too much salt results in potassium deficiency and water retention*
Spinach	*Too acidic*
Sugar	*Disturbs blood glucose levels, causing disturbed appetite and energy levels*
Tomatoes	*Too acidic*

As you can see, the choice of available foods on the Detox Programme is extensive, so there is absolutely no excuse to stray from the programme. If you choose to use only a small selection of the foods available you will still be able to follow an interesting and varied programme, and those that you do not eat you can save for next time.

ADDITIONAL INFORMATION ON FOOD

Portion sizes

The Detox Programme is very specifically named – it is a programme and not a diet. A portion is a heaped table-spoon. Each meal will include a combination of at least three portions of either rice, vegetables or miscellaneous foods. Each meal should be a full plate or bowl. If at any stage you get hungry you must eat something, especially in the first half of the programme as your body adjusts. You are likely to think you are eating more than you should, but this is normal and correct.

Balanced diet

Vegetables, fruit and rice provide a great source of carbo-hydrates and fibre, whilst fish, oil and nuts are good sources of protein and fats. You must make sure that at least two portions of foods such as olive oil, cashew nuts and oily fish are included every day or your programme will lack the necessary balance – you are not eating any of your normal fats, so adding (beneficial) oils is crucial. If you just eat vegetables, rice and fruit you will get tired and your detox process will slow down to a stop.

Calorie intake

The Detox Programme is not calorie counted, but calories are a good way of demonstrating how much you need to eat. Calories are a measure of the amount of energy in our food. The average woman should eat around 1600 calories per day and never go below 1000 calories, even when dieting. If the calorie intake is reduced below 1000 we are not providing sufficient energy for our bodies to operate and we go into starvation mode – our bodies store fat for times when it is needed, the metabolism slows down and we become weak and lethargic. It is imperative that during the programme you don't let your intake go below the recom-mended 1200 calories per day: the detox will only work if you keep all your organs and systems functioning healthily.

Cooking techniques

While on the Detox Programme you should try to cook your foods as little as possible. The less heat the food is subjected to, the more nutrients will remain. Obviously all fish dishes need to be cooked thoroughly, but cooked vegetables should always be eaten slightly crisp and *al dente*. Techniques such as light steaming, parboiling, microwaving, stir-frying or flash-frying and grilling are much preferable to boiling or slow cooking, which destroy both flavour and nutrients.

Using your imagination

You have an extensive list of individual fresh foods, and what you need to do now is start using your imagination. Just because the list contains lots of individual items doesn't mean that you cannot combine them to make many commonly used foods – without any processing, additives, preservatives etc. Here are some basic examples of what you can include if you use foods from the lists and a little imagination.

Hummus

Garlic, olive oil, sesame seed paste (tahini), lemon juice and chick peas are all on the list. In Chapter 5 you will find a recipe for turning these ingredients into the most delicious home-made hummus you have ever tasted. Hummus is good for late-night snacks and for satisfying emergency hunger pangs.

Salad dressings

Olive oil, sesame oil, cider vinegar, lime juice, wholegrain mustard and pepper are all on the list. Chapter 5 will offer you a refreshingly sharp dressing for your salads.

Entertaining

Having friends for supper is easy on the Detox Programme. Fish, olives, herbs and vegetables are all on the list, and a meal of grilled fish with a herb and olive crust on a bed of chargrilled vegetables drizzled with olive oil is a gastronomic treat at any time. There are so many other combinations among the recipes in Chapter 5 that your guests would find it hard to believe if you told them they were 'detoxing'.

ON TO THE NEXT STAGE

Now that you have the food basics we need to look at the body care basics and recipe suggestions. In later chapters we shall look at all the ways to enhance the programme further and to pamper yourself during the programme.

It is very important to carry out the body care section of the programme, as it is designed to enhance and speed up the detox process. The treatments enhance the programme because they complement everything that you will be doing for yourself during the next thirty days: Don't think they are a luxury just because they are nice – make sure you realise they are a necessity.

'My hair and fingernails have grown like wildfire, I've lost a lot of excess fluid so my legs feel lighter, my stomach is flat as a board. I feel squeaky-clean and vital.'

Kate, London

BODY CARE AND THE DETOX PROGRAMME

The Detox Programme is all you will ever need to keep your body in the best possible condition from within. The nutrients from the foods, the internal cleansing actions of the rice, lemon water, fluids and so on, the cleansing of the eliminatory organs, the supplements and 'everyday foods' will all provide a fully rounded internal cleanse. The Detox Programme is also the main and most important way to keep your body in the best possible condition from the outside. But there is much more to do to enhance the vitality of your body and mind through a daily and weekly body care routine.

When you start the Detox Programme, from Day 1 to Day 30 you must:

- Take a cold shower every morning
- Do dry skin brushing every morning
- Self massage every morning and evening
- Take thirty minutes' exercise every day
- Have ten minutes' relaxation every day
- Have five minutes of quality breathing every day
- Say five affirmations or do five visualisations ten times each every day
- Smile or laugh heartily every day

- Exfoliate every three days
- Take an Epsom salts bath every five days

'What I hadn't expected was that my skin would feel so soft – it glowed with health after only three weeks.'

S. Payne, London

THE DAILY TREATMENTS

Cold shower

An invigorating swim in a cool pool, sea or lake every morning would be an ideal scenario. The cold water will increase your circulation, tone your muscles and skin and give the lymph a jump start. But if you needed to include a long cool swim every day on the Detox Programme, alongside all your other new activities, you would soon find that you would be spending more time detoxing and less time living your life! The alternative takes two minutes and has all the benefits of the swim without having to leave your own home – just take a cold shower.

This may sound mad, but if you have ever taken a shower or bath in a place where there was no hot water you will remember that it was a most invigorating experience that actually left you considerably warmer than it would if you had taken a normal hot shower. Indeed, in hot weather it is more effective to take a shower that is lukewarm or at blood temperature rather than a cold shower; the latter will increase your circulation and warm you up rather than cool you down.

When bathing or showering in the mornings, simply turn the shower to cold just before you are ready to finish and let the icy-cold water run over your entire body for just one minute. Alternatively, when you have finished your bath you can turn on the cold tap as the bathwater is draining away, cup your hands under the water and splash it all over your body.

Dry skin brushing

This once-unheard-of process now bounces from every health article you read – and quite right too! Sloughing away dead skin cells helps remove any barriers to your skin 'breathing' efficiently. It clears the pores and improves the appearance of the skin – dead skin is dull and does not reflect light well, whereas healthy skin glows in normal light conditions. Brushing also stimulates the production of sebum, which in turn helps to improve the texture and tone of the skin.

Brushing improves blood and lymph circulation by stimulating muscle contraction. The improved lymph flow causes more efficient excretion of waste materials in the cells and interstitial fluids occurring in the spaces between organs and tissues. Clearing this area encourages more efficient cell production and renewal. Increasing the flow of interstitial fluid also causes excess fluids to drain and clear from the more troublesome areas of the hips and thighs. Pooling, water retention or oedema can be prevented with more efficient fluid and lymph flow.

Effective brushing

Now that you have plenty of excellent reasons to dry skin brush, the next step is to know how to do it effectively.

1. Take a natural bristle brush, a loofah, a dry flannel or mitt. The brush or flannel etc. should be firm but not hard, as you will be brushing your skin quite vigorously all over your body – the skin on your stomach, for instance, is softer than the skin on your shins or forearms. Do not wet or moisturise the skin, as this may cause dragging.

2. Undress to your underwear or, preferably, take all your clothes off. Stand or sit in a position that gives you access to all parts of your body – the edge of the bed with your feet up on pillows is quite good, or you can sit on the edge of the bath with one foot up on the toilet seat if it is close enough.

3. Start at your feet and systematically work up towards the top of your body. All strokes should be towards the heart – the heart is a wonderful machine for pumping the blood down and out to all parts of the body, but both blood and lymph need extra help to work against gravity to return through the system. If you brush away from the heart it may cause faintness or disrupt the normal flow. Each stroke should be long and firm. Place the brush/mitt on your ankle and firmly brush up to your knee, then repeat until you have covered the entire calf and shin several times. When you have completed the lower leg move up to the knee. The next set of strokes should run from the knee to the top of the thigh and over the buttocks.

4. Then brush both arms, from the wrist to the shoulder. The neck and shoulder area should be treated more gently as the flesh here is very delicate. Work from the top of your arm, up and over your shoulder and gently up your neck to the base of your skull.

5. When brushing your stomach, use gentle circular strokes in a clockwise direction. This will follow the flow in your intestines and will not disrupt any bowel functions.

6. You must only brush your face with a soft facial brush or flannel, as the skin here is very delicate and can be damaged if the brush is too hard.

The whole process should only take three or four minutes and afterwards you should feel invigorated. Your skin will tingle and you should feel quite warm as you will have stimulated and increased your circulation. After only a few sessions you will notice quite a difference in your skin – it feels smoother, with a softer texture, and the dry patches will have all disappeared. Just spend a little time each day and you will be pleasantly surprised.

Self massage

I could go on for days about how good massage is for everything! I have put a full description of its methods and benefits on pages 150 and 171, so I will limit what I say here to the more specific ways that massage can enhance the detox process. Everything we know about the benefits of massage is true for self massage. It would be wonderful if we could all have massage treatments every day of our lives, but it takes time and money and a lot of practitioners. Self massage avoids all those problems: it is cheap and can be done any time or anywhere. Since daily massage is required on the thirty-day programme, self massage is essential.

So why is massage so good for detox? This list is just for starters – there are many more beneficial effects:

- It warms and relaxes our muscles

- It relieves tension

- It helps to reduce stress

- It increases the blood circulation

- It increases lymph flow

- It helps to improve the immune system

- It helps the body eliminate excess fluids

- It helps the body eliminate waste products

- It improves the flow of interstitial fluid, improving the appearance of the skin, especially in areas prone to cellulite

- It lowers blood pressure

- It tones the muscles

- It tones the skin

- It is a passive workout for the whole body

Self massage techniques

Most normal massage strokes can be converted for self massage. As long as you observe the general rules of massage, even 'made up' strokes will be perfectly acceptable and effective.

- As with dry skin brushing, all massage strokes should be towards the heart, pushing the blood around the system in conjunction with the circulation and not against it

- All strokes should be done using either the flat hand (fingers together, palms down) or with the ends of the fingers (bunched together, no fingernails)

- All massage strokes should start lightly and slowly build to a firmer, more rapid pace

- The flesh should be warm and relaxed before any deeper strokes can be used. Working deeply on cold, tense flesh will feel unpleasant and cause bruising

- Massage should never be painful or sore, but massage that is too light is little better than a comforting stroke

- You should be relaxed when carrying out self massage as you need to work in some awkward positions and do not want to cause any twists or injuries

You should massage yourself every day during the Detox Programme, but as this can become time-consuming I have broken down the massage sequence into smaller elements. Try to do at least two of the elements every day to ensure that over each week you will get a full body treatment. Remember, take it slowly at first. Then, as your knowledge and confidence build, you will be able to make adjustments as necessary.

Where possible you should make sure that the room you are in is warm and quiet, perhaps with some relaxing or calming music. If the room is cold it is likely that you will not be totally relaxed, which will not result in the best massage.

You should use a massage oil, favourite cream or body lotion and apply just enough to allow your hands to work over the flesh firmly. If you use too much you will just slip over the skin, and if you use too little you may pull or 'burn' the skin. Reapply as necessary. If you apply too much, just wipe the excess on another part of the body until you need it later.

Face and neck sequence

Place the pads of your fingers together and press them on to your face quite firmly. Working together, circle both hands upwards, out and down, all over the surface of your face – remember to work the cheeks, forehead, nose, lips etc. Then relax your jawbone and let your mouth relax. Continue strokes down your neck and over the front of your chest in small and large circles.

Shoulder and arm sequence

Place your hand flat on to your lower arm. Keeping as much of your hand as possible on the arm, work in long, smooth, firm strokes from the base of the arm, up and over the shoulder. The pressure should be on the upward stroke, and released on the downward stroke. What you are doing is pushing the blood up towards the top of your arm.

Hand and wrist sequence

Place the thumb of your left hand on the knuckle of your right thumb. 'Drain' the blood and lymph from your knuckle to your wrist in long, smooth strokes. Repeat with all knuckles on that hand until you have 'drained' the entire hand and wrist. Firm pressure is required from the start to the end of each stroke. Do the same for your left hand.

Stomach and chest sequence

Place your hands flat on your stomach and massage both of them in large circles over the entire torso. The right hand should travel anticlockwise and the left hand clockwise, with firm strokes.

Lower back and spine sequence

Stand with your legs shoulder-width apart. Place your hands on your hips with the fingers in front and the thumbs on your back. Press your thumbs firmly into your spine and lower back and move in deep, firm circles. Cover as much of the spine area as possible.

Thigh and buttock sequence

Sit with your legs supported on the side of the bed or bath or with pillows underneath them. Working on one leg at a time, use flat hands to work in firm circles over the entire buttock and thigh area. Once the flesh becomes warm and slightly pink, clench your fist and continue with the firm circles. Work gently at first and build the pressure slowly.

Calf and foot sequence

Placing both hands flat on to the tops of your feet, brush them up towards your knees in long, firm strokes. Repeat rapidly several times. Move your hands to the back of your leg and press the flesh firmly, lifting it and pushing it alternately. Work the flesh backwards and forwards, taking care not to 'burn' it.

Exercise

This is one of the best ways to enhance the Detox Programme. It costs nothing, it can be done at any time of the day or night, even whilst you are doing everyday chores, and it can have many, many benefits. The Fitness Association in the UK issued a list of reasons why exercise was good for you, and the ones in *italics* are particularly relevant to the Detox Programme:

- Promotes increased stamina
- Relieves symptoms of menopause
- May help prevent heart disease
- Prevents osteoporosis
- Reduces the risk of breast cancer
- Lessens arthritis pain
- Controls cholesterol
- Burns fat
- *Speeds up metabolism*
- Alleviates PMT
- Improves neuromuscular (nerve and muscle) coordination
- Increases the body's ability to fight off infection
- Reduces the risk of glaucoma
- Decreases the risk of colon cancer
- Lowers blood pressure
- Reduces the risk of obesity
- Burns calories
- *Relieves constipation*
- Prevents endometriosis

- Helps you to stop smoking
- Relieves depression
- Releases anxiety
- Improves sexual performance
- Improves mental sharpness
- Improves concentration
- Improves outlook
- Reduces medical costs
- Increases job satisfaction
- Preserves muscle
- Preserves internal organs (liver, kidneys)
- Improves reaction time
- Increases range of motion
- *Improves cardiovascular fitness*
- *Increases energy*
- Reduces alcohol consumption
- Reduces stress
- *Enhances self-esteem*
- *Heightens sense of wellbeing*
- Increases IQ
- Enhances creativity
- Decreases job absenteeism
- Increases productivity
- Improves flexibility
- *Improves circulation*
- Increases mobility
- Improves memory
- Shortens recovery time after illness or injury
- Promotes a healthy back
- *Deepens sleep*
- *Lengthens life*

You should do at least thirty minutes' exercise every day during your Detox Programme. Not only will this help to keep you fit and toned, but it will also ensure that your metabolic rate does not decrease or your circulation become sluggish.

A little and often is much better than spending two hours every two weeks. The latter is likely to tire you out more quickly; also, you will not build up any benefit from your exercise as it happens too infrequently, which in turn will be discouraging and you may well give up. If you exercise for thirty minutes every day it doesn't interfere with your day too much, it's over before you get bored and you will notice the benefits after just a few days. So you are much more likely to get inspired and start extending thirty into forty minutes, until you build up to a level of exercise that naturally suits you and your lifestyle.

Getting started is the hardest part. Think about how your day works and how you can slip in the exercise without even noticing:

- If you normally start by going downstairs to get the post or to make breakfast, go up and down the stairs three times before you actually boil the kettle

- If you normally drive to pick up the children from school, then walk (it will do the children good, too)

- As you are cleaning the house you could jog whilst vacuuming or stretch for five minutes whilst dusting

- If you are going to be sitting in a meeting for several hours, go to the meeting room via the longest route and run up the stairs several times before sitting down

- In the evening whilst watching the television you can lift and lower your legs or tense and relax your stomach muscles several times

- When everyone is out of the house, put on some music and dance for thirty minutes – this feels great and is excellent exercise as well!

- Don't go out to the pub – go to a nightclub and dance

- Go rollerblading rather than walking on Sunday

- Don't watch the kids in the pool – get in there with them

- Sit in the bath and do stretches from side to side or

scissor your legs together and apart using the water as weights – but be careful not to splash too much!

Of course, the more traditional methods of exercise are still very valuable – joining a gymnasium, going to exercise classes, playing sport, jogging and so on. But if you have tried all these and not found your natural form of exercise, don't be discouraged. Set yourself a challenge to find the most unusual form of exercise you can, and do it for thirty minutes each day.

If you are the type of person who likes to follow sequences, get a video exercise tape of someone whom you like and admire and work with this, gradually building up the amount of time you spend until you can do the whole tape without blinking. If you are the type of person who likes to follow a set sequence, the following pages will take you through an elementary routine that you can do yourself.

Exercise sequence

1. Walk up and down ten steps or stairs for five minutes at a normal pace.

2. Stand with feet shoulder-width apart and alternately lift your left leg and left arm up and out to the side, then your right leg and right arm up and out to the side. Repeat ten times each side. NB: Keep your arms and knees slightly bent.

3. Standing in the same position as before, clasp your hands in front of your nose with your arms slightly bent. Keeping your shoulders relaxed, twist slowly from side to side. The stretch will gradually increase and you should end it when you can see directly behind yourself. Feel the stretch in your stomach and waist muscles. Repeat ten times each side.

4. Walk on the spot for five minutes, making sure that you bring each knee up to hip level. Swing your arms up and down in a marching style, bringing your hands up to shoulder height.

5. Walk on the spot for five minutes, bringing your knees up and out to the side to hip level. Clasp your hands in front of you with your forearms and elbows together, and as you step lift your arms and lower them. Don't let your arms drop below shoulder height.

6. Jog on the spot for five minutes without lifting your toes from the floor. You should be just lifting your heels up and down and wiggling your hips as much as possible.

7. Facing forward, twist your head slowly from side to side, looking over your right and left shoulders alternately. Hold the stretch for a moment, then release and look over the other shoulder.

8. Standing with feet shoulder-width apart, hold the back of an upright chair and lower your body until your knees are bent at 90 degrees. Hold this position for a count of five, then lift yourself slowly. Repeat fifteen times. Remember to clench your buttocks and thighs as you lift and lower your body.

9. Kneel on the floor with your hands shoulder-width apart and flat on the floor. Walk your hands forward so that you are supporting your body weight on your

hands and using your knees as a balance. Keeping your back straight, bend and lower your arms until your nose touches the floor, and then lift. Repeat ten times, slowly.

All these exercises, except the jogging, should be slow and deliberate. You should use your body weight as resistance to increase the effectiveness of the exercises. You can increase the number of repetitions as soon as you become comfortable with the programme – do them for as long as you wish, but for at least thirty minutes every day.

Whatever form of exercise you choose, you should treat it as something that you deserve and that enhances the Detox Programme. It is easy to think that exercise is hard work and a chore – something that both your mind and body have to endure – when actually both your body and mind love and need exercise in order to function efficiently.

Posture

Exercise is closely related to posture. We are all designed so that our internal organs have sufficient space to operate efficiently. If we change this spacing by putting on weight, losing weight, sitting with our bodies squashed or slumping whilst we eat, our organs need to compensate. This will lead to conditions like inefficient expansion of the lungs whilst breathing, lack of oxygen in the body, incorrect absorption of vital vitamins, minerals and foodstuffs, indigestion, poor circulation and headaches. More obvious physical effects occur as well: slouching shoulders, weak stomach muscles and a caved-in chest. Exercise will keep the body and its muscles in good condition to prevent any of these effects occurring, or will correct any that have already set in.

Breathing

Everyone knows how important oxygen, fresh air and good breathing are for us to survive. But if you ask anyone exactly how to breathe correctly or what effects good breathing has they will probably struggle for an explanation.

Breathing correctly is fundamental to survival, and even a momentary lack of the correct levels of oxygen in the body will result in serious damage and eventually death. Yet many of us continue to under-use the full capacity of our lungs and short-change our bodies of all the benefits that correct breathing will bring.

From early childhood we are told to 'stand up straight, stomachs in', and when we are told to take a deep breath we automatically inhale and raise our chests. But restricting movement of the stomach and abdomen means that we are limiting the area into which the lungs can expand, and so we develop the habit of only using a third of our lung capacity each time we inhale.

Balance of mind and body is also affected by breathing. If you are tense and stressed and your breathing is short and shallow you are less likely to be able to think straight, your movements become erratic and your balance is thrown.

Correct breathing is easy and more relaxing. Breathing exercises are simple and can be carried out whenever you feel it necessary.

To breathe correctly you simply relax your stomach muscles, inhale slowly through your nose and take in the air until it feels as if the base of your stomach is full of air. Then pause momentarily before exhaling through your mouth. Feeling the air 'in your stomach' shows that you have relaxed your diaphragm muscle, which means your lungs have fully expanded and you have inhaled to full capacity. This will feel strange at first, but it will soon become the normal way to breathe and you won't think about it any more.

Deeper breathing slows the heart rate and the pulse. Also, the deeper we breathe the more oxygen we inhale. All these are indications of improved and stronger health.

A simple breathing exercise

This is a good exercise to do when you feel stressed, if you cannot sleep or if you simply want to recharge your batteries.

1. Sit comfortably or lie down, supporting your lower back if necessary.

2. Place your hands on your stomach area with the fingertips just touching.

3. Start to breathe in through your nose very slowly to a count of four. As you inhale you should feel your stomach expand and your fingertips separate.

4. Hold your breath for four and exhale slowly through your mouth to a count of eight.

5. Repeat several times as required.

It will feel strange at first, as you are not accustomed to using your muscles to expand your stomach in this way. However, over a period of just a few minutes it will become more natural.

Continue this exercise for at least ten inward breaths and you should feel much more relaxed and 'centred'. Eventually you will not need to use your fingers to check that your stomach is expanding rather than your chest, and soon you will be able to carry out the exercise whilst going about your normal day-to-day business – not the lying down, but the controlled breathing! If you ever have difficulty in dropping off to sleep this is a far more effective way than the traditional 'counting sheep'. The chances are that you won't make it to ten and will probably be asleep by six.

Affirmations and visualisations

Here is a brilliant way of feeling good about yourself immediately, with long-term benefits as well. Feeling down in the dumps can be transformed into feeling positive and proactive in just a matter of moments. Once you have got into the habit of affirmations and visualisations, feeling depressed will become a thing of the past.

During the detox you can affirm your ability to complete the programme and you can visualise just how 'clean' you will be when you have finished. When you have completed the detox, when you are thinking about beginning – or just about any other time in your life – you can use affirmations and visualisations to help you.

You often hear people say, 'And if someone tells you this often enough, you really start to believe them.' That's all that affirmations are – telling yourself something, anything, often enough that you really believe it, and if you believe something it becomes real.

Affirmations don't have to be grand or extraordinary; they just have to help you. To start making affirmations you need to think about what your goal is, what you want to happen or what you want to do. It can be on any level: personal, job, home, relationship, money – anything. It is probably better to start with something small – giving up your job and living on a tropical island might be a little too adventurous for starters! And anyway, if you change something small it always leads to something bigger.

Affirmations must be positive and should be kept short. The sort of thing you may want to affirm during the detox would be:

- I have a healthy body

- I am happy with my body

- I am cleaning my body

- This is my month, I will enjoy looking after myself

- I deserve to indulge myself this month

- I am feeling great

- I am feeling energetic

- I have succeeded with my own personal detox

You get the idea ... Now all you have to do is repeat these to yourself or out loud. You should say them whenever they come into your mind; you can say all of them or you can say just one of them. As you are saying your affirmations you should give them positive energy, feel good about saying them and smile. You should believe that they are real and that they have come true or are coming true for you. If there is a time when you say your affirmations and you feel any doubt or negative feelings, immediately say them again and this time with all the positive belief that you can muster.

If you find it difficult to remember your affirmations, just jot them down on your 'to do' list, your shopping list or your diary. Then each time you see them, say them to yourself two or three times.

Affirmations are completely personal. No one needs to hear them or even know that you make them. The only rule is that they just have to be what you want:

- I deserve more money

- I am going to get a better job

- I am great

- I am fun to be with

- I am going to ask him/her out

- I will tell him/her that I don't agree

- I will have more time for myself

- I won't let them get to me

- I am successful in everything I do

Visualisations are very like affirmations, but you make mental pictures of whatever you want to happen. You need to create a clear picture of the object, person or situation in the way that you want it to be. Make the picture in the present and not the future: this way you can see things happening rather than waiting for them to happen. Include as many details as you can so that the image is as real as possible. As with affirmations you should bring this picture to mind as often as you can, keeping the thoughts that surround the picture positive and full of energy.

Visualisation should be a pleasant, uplifting process – not exhausting, or you will defeat the object. The more you visualise your situation, the more it becomes part of your life and closer to reality.

Affirmations and visualisations are ways to think and see yourself reaching your goals and achieving your own success in a personal way. When you have been doing them for a while you will notice subtle changes, and your friends and colleagues will keep saying how much more positive and 'up' you seem.

Relaxation

If you are fit and healthy and detoxed, relaxation can be a continual state. That is not to say that you will be so relaxed that you never do anything or you stop responding to outside stimulis, more that everything you do is done in a way that does not harm your body or put you under any unnecessary stress. You can be making a presentation to five hundred delegates at a conference but still remain relaxed, and you can stand in a queue at the supermarket with four impatient children and still remain relaxed. All you have to do is use some simple relaxation techniques.

Once you have combined affirmations and visualisations (see p.74) and correct breathing (see p.72), it is very easy to keep yourself in a permanent state of relaxation. This is not a permanent state of being 'laid back' or 'not caring', but a permanent state of being in control, calm and confident.

We have discussed breathing and what an important part it plays in staying relaxed. We have discussed visualisations and affirmations and how these can boost your confidence in achieving your goals. If you truly believe that you will get everything you want in life and you are 'centred and grounded' with regular deep breathing, then you will achieve true relaxation. Of course there are hurdles and hiccups along the way, but if the future holds all you desire then relaxation is natural.

A simple relaxation exercise

Practice makes perfect. The more you actively practise relaxation techniques the more easy they become and, as with the breathing exercises, you will soon be able to take yourself into deep relaxation at any time during the day or night. All you have to do is memorise this sequence or even record it onto a tape very slowly and play it to yourself as you are relaxing.

1. Find a quiet room, make sure you are warm and choose some music that is melodic and peaceful.

2. Lie down on the floor or sit comfortably in a chair.

3. Close your eyes and start to breathe deeply as described in the breathing exercise on p.73.

4. After breathing correctly for a couple of minutes you should find that your breathing has slowed down and you feel very natural.

5. When you inhale, imagine that the air you are breathing is warm and golden and is bathing your body in warm, golden, restful and positive light.

6. Now start to consider how your body is feeling. As you inhale start thinking about the feet and ankle area of your body. Are they tense? If so, relax them.

7. As you exhale, picture the air you breathe out to be the old, stagnant air and the air you breathe in to be the new, fresh air.

8. Think of your calves and knees. Picture the warm air travelling through any tense muscles, bathing them in light. Exhale the stale air.

9. Picture your knee joints and your upper leg area. Breathe deeply and relax.

10. Feel the air being breathed into the groin area, relaxing the tension and soothing the pelvis. Breathe out the bad air.

11. See the golden light swirling around your stomach

and abdomen, cleansing and uplifting your centre of emotion and spirit.

12. Watch the light thread its way between each and every rib, filling your lungs and chest cavity with warm, expanding air.

13. Watch each and every finger fill with golden light which spreads through your fingers and lower arms.

14. Breathe in the energy into your shoulders and base of your neck. Feel your neck relax and melt into the floor or back of the chair and up into the base of your skull.

15. The light may now travel into the root of each and every hair follicle, making your scalp feel invigorated and tingling.

16. Each time you exhale you are breathing out waste. Each time you breathe in you are breathing in new life.

17. When you have renewed the life inside your body, look to see where the source of your new breath and new light is coming from.

18. With your eyes still closed, look above you and see the beam of light coming down towards your body – see it feeding into your abdomen. You are connected to this light and you can take as much as you wish.

19. Breathe deeply and inhale all you need.

20. When you are ready you can start to think about bringing your consciousness back into your own body and into the room you are in.

21. Open your eyes slowly. If you are lying on the floor or bed, roll over on to your side and wait a few moments before pushing yourself up to a sitting and then a standing position.

22. You should now feel totally relaxed and invigorated – well done!

LESS REGULAR TREATMENTS

Exfoliation

Dry skin brushing is just as it sounds – dry! This means it is quick and convenient if you are including it in your morning routine before the children need taking to nursery or you have to dash off to work, or when you simply want a great wake-up energy booster. Exfoliation has all the benefits of the brushing technique but can be included in the more relaxing, more tranquil or even indulgent times of the Detox Programme. Just make sure you carry it out once every three days while on the programme. Exfoliation needs water and some form of home-made or cosmetic exfoliant. This process is generally more gentle on the skin than dry brushing and can therefore be used on the face and any other delicate areas that might find dry brushing a little too harsh. Exfoliating products are widely available in all price ranges and are usually combined with wonderful-smelling creams or gels. However, if you don't wish to spend money on an exfoliating scrub you can easily make your own.

Home-made exfoliating mix

Enough for one bath/scrub

- 1 tablespoon salt flakes (use ordinary household salt if your skin is delicate or you want a less rigorous product)

- 2 tablespoons vegetable or seed oil (olive, sunflower, sesame etc.)

- 1 tablespoon honey

Place all the ingredients in a plastic bowl and mix them together until you have a runny paste. Dip the ends of your fingers into the pot and scoop about a teaspoon of the mix out each time. Rub this all over the body and apply more when required. (The salt is the exfoliant and the oil and honey will help to moisturise the flesh.)

Alternatively you can turn your favourite body oil into an exfoliant by simply adding the salt to a small amount of your chosen product and then using as described below.

You can exfoliate in the bath or shower, but unless you have a palatial shower you may find that the cream has been washed off before you get the chance to benefit from its exfoliating properties! Ideally you should exfoliate during a nice relaxing bath. Here's how.

Run a bath and put a few drops of your favourite bath oil or foam into the water. Get in and relax. Allow at least ten minutes before you start to exfoliate, as this will give you time to relax and your skin time to soften in the water.

There are now two options, of which this is the first.

Get out of the bath, making sure the bathroom is still nice and warm, and gently rub your exfoliating cream or home-made exfoliant in firm circles, both large and small, all over your body. Pay special attention to any areas of hard skin – heels, knees, elbows etc. – and rub as hard as you find comfortable. The whole process should take about three or four minutes. When you have completed the rub, get back into the bath and carry on the circular rubbing until all the cream has been washed off into the bathwater. Get out of the bath and then rub yourself dry with a towel (not one that has been rinsed in fabric conditioner, as this will increase its absorbency and carry on the exfoliating process as you are drying yourself). Once you are dry, apply a good moisturiser or body oil all over your body and stay warm. Going to bed with a book or for an early night is a good next move.

Now for the second option. Stay in the bath and, lifting each limb in turn above the surface of the water, exfoliate as described above, in firm circles both large and small. As you finish each limb lower it back into the water and continue to work the flesh until all the cream has been washed away. The only area that may get neglected if you are using this method is the buttocks, but you can do them by kneeling up in the bath. Towel yourself dry as above, and then moisturise and keep warm in the same way.

Epsom salts baths

Magnesium is an essential requirement for nearly all our cellular activity. It can be found in high concentration in Epsom salts, which are pure magnesium, and bathing in

Epsom salts allows the skin to absorb it. As well as the skin absorbing the magnesium the magnesium will absorb or 'draw' toxins from the body, so it is likely that you will 'glow' with perspiration for a while after your bath. This will not be quite a sweat unless you wrap up really warm! It is more likely to feel as if you are in a very humid room. It is very important to keep warm – not only to increase the effect of the magnesium but also to prevent yourself catching a chill. Epsom salts baths will improve your circulation and speed up the elimination of toxins. You should take one every five days while on the programme

An Epsom salts bath can also be extremely relaxing and warming, helping to soothe aching joints and muscles. Taken at bedtime it will almost certainly guarantee your deepest night's sleep ever!

To make the ideal Epsom salts bath

Run a deep bath that is warm enough to sit in comfortably for ten or fifteen minutes without going cold. Pour about 2lb (1kg) (yes, 2lb! It is a lot but you need this much to get the best effect) of Epsom salts (available from most chemists or health food stores) into your bath and stir until it has all dissolved. Get into the bath and have ready a loofah glove or massage mitt.

Sit in the bath for at least five minutes before you start to massage your body. Then start massaging with slow, gentle strokes, and as you get more used to this make the strokes more vigorous. It is likely that you will feel very warm quite quickly as the magnesium has this effect. If this happens, slow down your massage and just let the Epsom salts work on you as you relax.

When you get out of the bath pat yourself dry and then wrap up warmly for the next hour or so. Ideally the bath should be taken in the evening just before you go to bed, which will keep you warm for many hours. Alternatively you can take the bath during the day, then wrap up in a quilt or blanket and sit and watch an old movie!

Don't be surprised if you feel quite tired after an Epsom salts bath, as it will be having quite a major effect on your internal systems – all for the good. For best results you should take an Epsom salts bath every three days during the Detox Programme, but don't take one if you suffer from any skin condition or have any cuts or grazes.

Now that you are aware of all the body care treatments that are a required part of the Detox Programme you can plan the timing of your own programme and decide exactly when to start. On the following four pages there is a form for daily completion. Make sure that you tick each box every day, and then you can be sure that nothing has been missed. You may want to photocopy the chart first.

Daily food and activity checklist

	1	2	3	4	5	6	7	8
Cold shower/bath	☐	☐	☐	☐	☐	☐	☐	☐
Dry skin brushing	☐	☐	☐	☐	☐	☐	☐	☐
Moisturising	☐	☐	☐	☐	☐	☐	☐	☐
Hot lemon and water	☐	☐	☐	☐	☐	☐	☐	☐
Fruit	☐	☐	☐	☐	☐	☐	☐	☐
Goat's/sheep's yoghurt	☐	☐	☐	☐	☐	☐	☐	☐
Goat's/sheep's cheese	☐	☐	☐	☐	☐	☐	☐	☐
Nuts	☐	☐	☐	☐	☐	☐	☐	☐
Seeds/pulses/beans	☐	☐	☐	☐	☐	☐	☐	☐
Brown rice	☐	☐	☐	☐	☐	☐	☐	☐
Salads	☐	☐	☐	☐	☐	☐	☐	☐
Fish (optional)	☐	☐	☐	☐	☐	☐	☐	☐
3 pints (1.7 litres) water	☐	☐	☐	☐	☐	☐	☐	☐
Herbal teas	☐	☐	☐	☐	☐	☐	☐	☐
Liver tonic x 2	☐	☐	☐	☐	☐	☐	☐	☐
Kidney tonic x 2	☐	☐	☐	☐	☐	☐	☐	☐
30 minutes' exercise	☐	☐	☐	☐	☐	☐	☐	☐
10 minutes' total relaxation	☐	☐	☐	☐	☐	☐	☐	☐
5 minutes' 'quality' breathing	☐	☐	☐	☐	☐	☐	☐	☐
5 affirmations or visualisations repeated 10 times each	☐	☐	☐	☐	☐	☐	☐	☐
Smile or laugh heartily	☐	☐	☐	☐	☐	☐	☐	☐
Exfoliation every third day	☐	☐	☐	☐	☐	☐	☐	☐
Epsom salts bath 6 times during Detox Programme	☐	☐	☐	☐	☐	☐	☐	☐
Treatment every 4 days: aroma, massage, reflex etc. (optional)	☐	☐	☐	☐	☐	☐	☐	☐

Daily food and activity checklist

	9	10	11	12	13	14	15	16
Cold shower/bath	☐	☐	☐	☐	☐	☐	☐	☐
Dry skin brushing	☐	☐	☐	☐	☐	☐	☐	☐
Moisturising	☐	☐	☐	☐	☐	☐	☐	☐
Hot lemon and water	☐	☐	☐	☐	☐	☐	☐	☐
Fruit	☐	☐	☐	☐	☐	☐	☐	☐
Goat's/sheep's yoghurt	☐	☐	☐	☐	☐	☐	☐	☐
Goat's/sheep's cheese	☐	☐	☐	☐	☐	☐	☐	☐
Nuts	☐	☐	☐	☐	☐	☐	☐	☐
Seeds/pulses/beans	☐	☐	☐	☐	☐	☐	☐	☐
Brown rice	☐	☐	☐	☐	☐	☐	☐	☐
Salads	☐	☐	☐	☐	☐	☐	☐	☐
Fish (optional)	☐	☐	☐	☐	☐	☐	☐	☐
3 pints (1.7 litres) water	☐	☐	☐	☐	☐	☐	☐	☐
Herbal teas	☐	☐	☐	☐	☐	☐	☐	☐
Liver tonic x 2	☐	☐	☐	☐	☐	☐	☐	☐
Kidney tonic x 2	☐	☐	☐	☐	☐	☐	☐	☐
30 minutes' exercise	☐	☐	☐	☐	☐	☐	☐	☐
10 minutes' total relaxation	☐	☐	☐	☐	☐	☐	☐	☐
5 minutes' 'quality' breathing	☐	☐	☐	☐	☐	☐	☐	☐
5 affirmations or visualisations repeated 10 times each	☐	☐	☐	☐	☐	☐	☐	☐
Smile or laugh heartily	☐	☐	☐	☐	☐	☐	☐	☐
Exfoliation every third day	☐	☐	☐	☐	☐	☐	☐	☐
Epsom salts bath 6 times during Detox Programme	☐	☐	☐	☐	☐	☐	☐	☐
Treatment every 4 days: aroma, massage, reflex etc. (optional)	☐	☐	☐	☐	☐	☐	☐	☐

Daily food and activity checklist

	17	18	19	20	21	22	23	24
Cold shower/bath	☐	☐	☐	☐	☐	☐	☐	☐
Dry skin brushing	☐	☐	☐	☐	☐	☐	☐	☐
Moisturising	☐	☐	☐	☐	☐	☐	☐	☐
Hot lemon and water	☐	☐	☐	☐	☐	☐	☐	☐
Fruit	☐	☐	☐	☐	☐	☐	☐	☐
Goat's/sheep's yoghurt	☐	☐	☐	☐	☐	☐	☐	☐
Goat's/sheep's cheese	☐	☐	☐	☐	☐	☐	☐	☐
Nuts	☐	☐	☐	☐	☐	☐	☐	☐
Seeds/pulses/beans	☐	☐	☐	☐	☐	☐	☐	☐
Brown rice	☐	☐	☐	☐	☐	☐	☐	☐
Salads	☐	☐	☐	☐	☐	☐	☐	☐
Fish (optional)	☐	☐	☐	☐	☐	☐	☐	☐
3 pints (1.7 litres) water	☐	☐	☐	☐	☐	☐	☐	☐
Herbal teas	☐	☐	☐	☐	☐	☐	☐	☐
Liver tonic x 2	☐	☐	☐	☐	☐	☐	☐	☐
Kidney tonic x 2	☐	☐	☐	☐	☐	☐	☐	☐
30 minutes' exercise	☐	☐	☐	☐	☐	☐	☐	☐
10 minutes' total relaxation	☐	☐	☐	☐	☐	☐	☐	☐
5 minutes' 'quality' breathing	☐	☐	☐	☐	☐	☐	☐	☐
5 affirmations or visualisations repeated 10 times each	☐	☐	☐	☐	☐	☐	☐	☐
Smile or laugh heartily	☐	☐	☐	☐	☐	☐	☐	☐
Exfoliation every third day	☐	☐	☐	☐	☐	☐	☐	☐
Epsom salts bath 6 times during Detox Programme	☐	☐	☐	☐	☐	☐	☐	☐
Treatment every 4 days: aroma, massage, reflex etc. (optional)	☐	☐	☐	☐	☐	☐	☐	☐

Daily food and activity checklist

	25	26	27	28	29	30
Cold shower/bath	☐	☐	☐	☐	☐	☐
Dry skin brushing	☐	☐	☐	☐	☐	☐
Moisturising	☐	☐	☐	☐	☐	☐
Hot lemon and water	☐	☐	☐	☐	☐	☐
Fruit	☐	☐	☐	☐	☐	☐
Goat's/sheep's yoghurt	☐	☐	☐	☐	☐	☐
Goat's/sheep's cheese	☐	☐	☐	☐	☐	☐
Nuts	☐	☐	☐	☐	☐	☐
Seeds/pulses/beans	☐	☐	☐	☐	☐	☐
Brown rice	☐	☐	☐	☐	☐	☐
Salads	☐	☐	☐	☐	☐	☐
Fish (optional)	☐	☐	☐	☐	☐	☐
3 pints (1.7 litres) water	☐	☐	☐	☐	☐	☐
Herbal teas	☐	☐	☐	☐	☐	☐
Liver tonic x 2	☐	☐	☐	☐	☐	☐
Kidney tonic x 2	☐	☐	☐	☐	☐	☐
30 minutes' exercise	☐	☐	☐	☐	☐	☐
10 minutes' total relaxation	☐	☐	☐	☐	☐	☐
5 minutes' 'quality' breathing	☐	☐	☐	☐	☐	☐
5 affirmations or visualisations repeated 10 times each	☐	☐	☐	☐	☐	☐
Smile or laugh heartily	☐	☐	☐	☐	☐	☐
Exfoliation every third day	☐	☐	☐	☐	☐	☐
Epsom salts bath 6 times during Detox Programme	☐	☐	☐	☐	☐	☐
Treatment every 4 days: aroma, massage, reflex etc. (optional)	☐	☐	☐	☐	☐	☐

The thirty-day programme – trouble-shooting and common side-effects

Problem/condition	Reason/solution
Fuzzy tongue	This is a normal sign that the body is getting rid of toxins. Rinse your mouth each morning with lemon water or scrape your tongue with a toothbrush until it feels cleaner. During the day you can chew on parsley if you find that the garlic is affecting your breath.
Headache	Detoxing means you will be 'coming off' some chemicals such as caffeine, alcohol or sugar. This may cause mild headaches as your body adjusts and is quite normal. Drinking fluids, taking rest and relaxation will help relieve the discomfort.
Constipation	Change in diet may sometimes lead to mild constipation. This should not last for more than a few days. Eat plenty of rice and raw vegetables and check that you are not eating too much cheese. You will soon find your bowel movements becoming healthy and regular.
Tiredness/lethargy	When your body first embarks on the detox it will be hard work on the internal organs and can be tiring. This will only last for a few days as you go through your 'healing crisis', and after that you will feel very energetic. If you feel tired later on during the programme you should check that you are eating enough – too little food can be very depleting.
Flu-like symptoms	Again, these can be due to the expected starting 'changes' during the programme and are normal in the first week or so. If you

Problem/condition	Reason/solution
	feel any of these symptoms after the first ten days look at the quantities you are eating and check that they are enough. Also look at how much you are exercising – you may be doing too much too soon.
Loose bowels	During the first three weeks of the programme your bowel movements will be loose. This is a result of the increased intake of fibre, the rice and the body cleaning out all its waste. This is normal and shows that the detox is working.
Nausea	This is not common and should be treated with caution. If you feel nauseous check you are eating enough and that your fluid intake is sufficient. Rest and relax, and don't exercise for that day.
Irritability	This is common. Try to do some breathing exercises or some actual exercise. Your body is going through some major changes and you should try to accommodate them as much as possible. It is just an indication that the bad is being cleared out!
Increased bowel movements	As with loose bowel movements, this is quite normal on the Detox Programme. It is likely that you will be making at least two movements a day – a sign that your body is processing foods efficiently and effectively.
Coloured urine	When you take vitamin supplements your urine is likely to change to a bright yellow/orange colour, and when you drink freshly juiced fruit or vegetables your urine will also change colour depending on the fruit or vegetable chosen – beetroot will turn it pink!

Problem/condition	Reason/solution
Spots	The skin is the body's biggest organ of elimination, so spots are very common during detox. You can reduce the risk of them if you drink lots of fluid and plenty of herbal teas that are diuretic (make you pass water) such as dandelion or fennel.
Change in skin tone	The efficiency of your circulation is greatly increased during the Detox Programme. This can lead to temporary 'rosy cheeks' or a 'glow', which will settle as your body adapts to the programme.
Runny nose or eyes, or sinus congestion	During the early stages of the programme it is likely that you may experience a slightly runny or blocked nose. This simply indicates that your body is clearing out or balancing your own fluid production, and the symptoms will only last a couple of days at most.

Stages of the thirty-day Detox Programme

	Energy	Skin	Fitness	Detox status
Day 1	Normal levels, no change	No change – normal dull, lifeless complexion	No change	In need of detox!
Day 3	Normal to lower as body experiences changes and detox organs begin to work harder	No real change, but dry skin brushing has begun to eliminate dead skin and pores begin to breathe	Possibly feeling slightly bloated as body gets used to extra water. Muscles may be aching from exercise	Enjoying the new regime. Realising how much you have neglected yourself recently
Day 5	Starting to feel different, not so tired last thing at night	More colour due to improved circulation, smoother due to massage and moisturisation	Muscle tone feels good but probably doesn't look very different. Stomach flatter	Going through the detox change. Things are beginning to happen!
Week 1	Feeling good, more vital and much more alert	Good colour but may have spots on face or elsewhere on body	Feeling good and leaner. Getting the exercise bug and seeing how body shape is changing in response to your efforts. Possible weight gain due to fat converting to muscle	First week successfully completed. Well done! Feeling more cleansed and more alert
Week 2	Lots of energy, not tired at night. Feeling fresh on waking and alert all day long	Smooth all over, skin positively glowing by now and any spots have cleared away	Clearer body lines, enjoying regular exercise, not exhausted and no muscle aches – feeling fit	Energy high, skin good, body fit. Feeling 'flushed out' and that you are getting full benefits and goodness from the food you eat
Week 3	Getting used to lots of energy. Feeling energetic is now normal	Smooth, good tone due to exercise. No dry patches, and great colour and warm glow	Probable weight loss. Good figure, flat stomach. Muscle definition at tops of arms, knees, stomach etc.	Energy reaches a high. You can feel that your insides are now nearly totally cleansed and your body is working on your behalf
Week 4	High energy is expected. You are now planning ahead, taking into account your increased energy levels	Looks and feels great	Regular exercise – no problem. Body in great shape and tone	Feel on top of the world, cleansed totally inside and out. Well done!

5

Recipes and Eating Suggestions

There are many recipes that can be used on the Detox Programme, and here are just a few to start you off. Remember to use your imagination and to experiment – there will be meals that you make and choose not to do again, but there will also be meals that you create that will become a staple part of your eating programme long after you have finished the detox.

The recipes and eating suggestions in this chapter are broken down into:

- Breakfasts

- Snacks

- Normal light meals, salads or side dishes

- Main courses

- Desserts

- Entertaining on the Detox Programme

- Logistical problems you may encounter whilst eating out on the Detox Programme, and solutions

BREAKFASTS

MUESLI

Sheep's yoghurt
Sunflower seeds
Sesame seeds
Pumpkin seeds
Dried apricots, chopped

Pour the yoghurt into a cereal bowl. Mix together the seeds and apricots and sprinkle over the top of the yoghurt. You can vary the quantities and proportions to suit your taste.

PEARS AND YOGHURT

1 pear
Apple juice
Goat's yoghurt

Peel the pear and place it in a pan with some apple juice and water. Bring to the boil and simmer until the pear has softened. Place the pear in a breakfast bowl and pour goat's yoghurt over it.

DETOX KEDGEREE

Smoked haddock (undyed)
Milk (rice, soya or goat's)
Brown rice, cooked
1 teaspoon olive oil
Goat's yoghurt
Cayenne pepper *or* parsley, chopped

(continues)

Place the fish in a pan and cover with milk. Simmer until the fish is soft and can be easily flaked. Remove the fish from the milk and drain. Flake the fish and mix it with the cooked brown rice and olive oil. Place a spoonful of yoghurt on top and sprinkle with the cayenne pepper or parsley.

FRUIT SALAD

A mixture of your favourite fruits, chopped into cubes
Apple juice
Juice of 1 fresh lime

Mix the cubed fruit and cover with apple juice. Pour the lime juice over the top and serve.

SNACKS

Whilst you are on the Detox Programme you should never be really hungry – if you are, either you are not eating enough or you have left a long time between meals. There are also times when you might like a light snack between meals. Obviously any of the dishes below can be made in smaller quantities, or you can eat any of the ingredients individually. Here are some other ideas for snacks.

POPCORN

Buy a packet as usual, but instead of making your popcorn in butter substitute olive oil. When the corn is ready you can add further flavour by tossing the warm kernels in a mixture of herbs.

RICE CAKES

These should be in the larder at home as an emergency snack. Make sure you buy the non-salted version, and have a selection of plain and sesame seed cakes to vary the flavour.

NUTS AND SEEDS

Make up a bag of mixed nuts and seeds to taste; you can also add chopped dried fruit for a little extra flavour. These are great, as they are small and will last in your handbag or desk for at least a week.

HOME-MADE HUMMUS

6 oz/175 g/1 cup dried chick peas *or* 1 can cooked chick peas
4 oz/110 g/$\frac{1}{2}$ cup tahini
Juice of 3 lemons
3 cloves garlic
4 fl oz/110 ml/$\frac{1}{2}$ cup olive oil

If using dried chick peas cook until tender (about an hour). If using canned, drain the brine thoroughly. Put the tahini, lemon juice, garlic and olive oil in a blender and mix thoroughly. Add the chick peas and blend until a thick paste is formed. You can add water to loosen the consistency, oil to make it more creamy, or more garlic and lemon to suit your taste.

NORMAL LIGHT MEALS, SALADS OR SIDE DISHES

All the following recipes are suitable for everyday meals, salads or side dishes. They are quite simple and straightforward and should take no more than ten minutes to prepare, assuming the rice is already cooked. It is a good idea to cook enough rice for two or three meals rather than each time you eat, as this will save time on preparation.

When oily fish such as tuna, mackerel or sardines are listed use fresh where possible, but canned versions are acceptable if they are in olive oil, vegetable oil or spring water. Don't use canned fish in brine, however, as the salt content is far too high. Remember: fresh is best.

When fruit or vegetables are listed, you must only use fresh produce. If it is not in season choose an available alternative to suit your taste – there really is no excuse for canned fruit or vegetables except canned tomatoes, and they are not on the food lists for the Detox Programme.

Unless stated, the recipes are for one. But each meal must be a plate or bowl *full*, so don't restrict your portion size. As the food is all fresh it will generally keep until the next meal without dressings, so make more rather than less – you should not be hungry on the Detox Programme.

CRUNCHY RED COLESLAW

Equal quantities to taste of:
Radishes, chopped
Red pepper, shredded
Cucumber, sliced in thin strips

Carrot, grated
Red cabbage, thinly sliced
Plus:
Smoked mackerel – a single fillet should be sufficient
Fresh coriander
Dressing:
1 tablespoon olive oil
1 teaspoon black pepper
1 dessertspoon lime juice

Mix all the shredded vegetables together and place in a large soup bowl. Mix the olive oil, black pepper and lime juice together and stir into the vegetables. Slice the mackerel fillet in strips and lay them on top of the coleslaw. Chop the fresh coriander and sprinkle it over the fish.

Serve with a *small* glass of apple juice.

GREEK POTATO

1 large potato
1 chunk cucumber
1 chunk ewe's Feta cheese
1 dessertspoon sesame oil
Fresh basil, chopped

Bake the potato until soft in the centre and crisp on the outside – you can start it off in the microwave and then crisp it in the oven on a baking tray for the final 20 minutes. Pre-heat the grill. Cube the cucumber and Feta and mix together. When the potato is ready, split it open and fork into the flesh the sesame oil and chopped basil, then push the flesh back into the skins and spoon the Feta/cucumber mixture on top. Place the whole dish under the grill until some of the Feta begins to melt.

Serve on a bed of mixed lettuce accompanied by a *small* glass of mineral water.

ROAST FENNEL WITH TUNA

1 portion brown rice

1 tablespoon olive oil

1 fennel bulb

1 portion cooked fresh tuna *or* tuna strips *or* canned tuna in spring water

Fresh sweetcorn *or* mini corn on the cobs

Juice of 1 lime

Fresh coriander, chopped

Freshly ground black pepper

Whilst boiling the rice, pre-heat the oven to 220°C (425°F/gas 7) pour the olive oil into a roasting tin and heat it in the oven. Slice the fennel bulb in half vertically, and when the oil is hot place the bulb cut side down in the roasting tin. Roast for 5 minutes and then turn and continue to roast until the bulb is slightly browned and soft in the middle. Flake the cooked tuna. When the rice is cooked, mix it with the flaked tuna and the raw sweetcorn. Toss with the lime juice, olive oil from the roasting tin and chopped coriander and place on a dinner plate. When the fennel is ready, place both halves on the bed of rice and tuna.

Serve with a grinding of black pepper.

Spicy courgette (zucchini) grill

Brown rice, cooked
1 large courgette (zucchini)
$\frac{1}{2}$ red bell pepper
$\frac{1}{2}$ green bell pepper
1 chunk ewe's Feta cheese, sliced
Chilli powder

Pre-heat the grill. Place a hearty serving of rice in the bottom of a heatproof bowl. Slice the courgette and cook it in the microwave for 3 minutes so that it is still crunchy. Shred the peppers and mix with the cooked courgette. Put the courgette mix on the rice and cover with slices of Feta. Place the whole bowl under the grill and toast until the cheese has browned on top.

Sprinkle with ground chilli powder (mild if preferred) before serving.

Fennel potato salad

1 portion new potatoes
1 red onion, chopped
1 fennel bulb, chopped
Olive oil
1 tablespoon pine nuts
1 portion cooked prawns
Lemon juice

Boil the new potatoes until nearly cooked, then drain and slice each potato in half. Fry the chopped onion and fennel bulb in the olive oil until translucent. Add the potato halves and fry until everything is slightly browned. Whilst browning the vegetables, lightly toast the pine nuts. When the vegetables have 2 minutes to go, add the prawns and the pine nuts and toss the whole salad together.

Serve with a drizzle of fresh lemon juice.

TUNA JACKET

1 large potato
Olive oil
1 portion tuna
2 small chicory bulbs, sliced
Balsamic vinegar

Bake the potato until soft. Pre-heat the grill. Drizzle a little olive oil over a piece of fresh tuna and grill it. Place strips of sliced chicory under the grill for the last few minutes of grilling. Make a dressing from 2 teaspoons of olive oil and balsamic vinegar to taste. Serve the tuna with the jacket potato and pour the dressing over the fish. You can also mix some of the dressing with the potato if you like.

Serve with a *small* glass of water.

NUT SALAD

2 tablespoons cashew nuts
2 tablespoons pine nuts
1 beetroot, cooked and chopped
Lettuce, shredded
2 tablespoons chopped fresh coriander leaves
Cucumber, chopped
Fennel bulb, chopped
Green bell pepper, chopped

4 tablespoons nut oil *or* olive oil
Juice of $\frac{1}{2}$ lemon

Toss all the ingredients together and serve. Alternatively you can serve the salad on top of a bed of brown rice or as an accompaniment to any of the main course dishes.

SARDINES WITH APRICOTS

1 portion brown rice
Fresh *or* canned sardines
1 portion soft goat's *or* sheep's cheese
5–6 dried apricots, soaked
$\frac{1}{2}$ green bell pepper
Nut oil (walnut, pistachio or hazelnut)
Lemon juice

Boil enough short grain brown rice to fill a large bowl. If using fresh sardines, grill them. Flake and bone the fish, fresh or canned, and mix into the rice. Cube the cheese and add to the mixture. Dice the apricots and add these too. Dice the green pepper and add. Dress with a blend of your chosen nut oil and lemon juice.

THAI CARROT SOUP

Carrots
Vegetable stock cube (from a health food shop, not the normal
  vegetable stock cubes as these contain preservatives and additives)
Lemon grass
1 chilli
Goat's *or* sheep's yoghurt
Fresh coriander, chopped

Boil the carrots in water with the stock cube, the lemon grass and the chilli. When the carrots are soft, remove the pan from the heat and drain. Keep the water but discard the lemon grass and chilli. Mash the carrots or put them in a blender until you have a smooth purée. Add some of the yoghurt and remaining stock water to get a soup-like consistency as thick or thin as you like. Reheat the soup and serve with a swirl of yoghurt and topped with the chopped coriander.

GINGER VEGETABLES

1 large portion mixed swede and carrots
1 small portion beetroot
4 tablespoons water
1 teaspoon crushed fresh ginger
1 tablespoon grated hard goat's cheese

Pre-heat the oven to 180°C/350°F/gas 4. Slice the vegetables into thin strips. Place them in a large ovenproof dish, stir in the water and ginger, and sprinkle cheese over the top. Bake slowly for about 50 minutes or until the vegetables are tender. Serve with more fresh ginger and coriander sprinkled on top.

ROAST BEETROOT

2 medium beetroot
Olive oil *or* nut oil
Fresh thyme, finely chopped
Lemon juice

Pre-heat the oven to 220°C/425°F/gas 7. Wash the beet-root. Mix the oil and thyme to make a dressing and roll the beetroot in it. Roast for about 1 hour, until tender. Remove from the oven, squeeze the lemon juice over the beetroot, reheat for 10 minutes and serve as you would jacket potatoes – perhaps with some Feta cheese crumbled over the top.

THREE BEAN SALAD

3 oz/90 g/$\frac{1}{2}$ cup kidney beans
3 oz/90 g/$\frac{1}{2}$ cup chick peas
3 oz/90 g/$\frac{1}{2}$ cup butter beans
1 red onion
1 clove garlic
3 tablespoons olive oil
Juice of $\frac{1}{2}$ lemon

Follow the general guidelines for bean soaking (usually overnight) and cooking on the packet or box, then drain and boil together until tender (1 hour). Alternatively, use ready-cooked beans canned in water or oil. Slice the onion finely and chop the garlic. Put all the ingredients into a medium bowl, toss lightly and leave in the fridge for at least 1 hour before serving.

MAIN COURSES

These dishes are slightly more complicated and will prob-ably need thirty minutes' preparation. All of them would be very suitable for entertaining at home, and of course they are also great for something different for your own main meals.

OVEN-BAKED STUFFED PEPPERS

1 red bell pepper
Creamed/soft goat's cheese
Basil leaves, chopped
1 clove garlic, finely sliced
Brown rice, cooked
Olive oil
To serve:
Assorted lettuce leaves
Cucumber
Olive oil
Lemon juice
Sesame seeds, regular or ready toasted

Slice the pepper in two vertically, remove the seeds and place on a baking tray in a medium oven (180°C/350°F/ gas 4) for 10 minutes to soften. Mix together the cheese, basil, garlic and rice. Stuff the peppers with this mixture and drizzle olive oil over them. Bake in the oven for a further 20 minutes or until ready.

Serve with a large salad of lettuce and cucumber in an oil and lemon juice dressing sprinkled with toasted sesame seeds.

SALMON WITH WATERCRESS

1 salmon steak *or* fillet
1 large portion watercress
Small piece red cabbage, shredded
$\frac{1}{2}$ red onion, sliced
Black olives
Small piece ewe's Feta cheese
Lime juice
Olive oil

Grill the salmon until slightly browned on top but still moist in the centre. Place some watercress on a dinner plate, lightly sprinkle red cabbage on top and then the onion. Scatter with the olives and the cheese, roughly crumbled. Place the salmon on top and dress with lime juice and olive oil.

Serve with a *small* glass of chilled apple juice.

NUTTY MONKFISH

Spring onions (scallions), sliced

10 cloves garlic

Cayenne pepper

3 tablespoons walnut oil

1 piece monkfish, cubed

$\frac{1}{2}$ red bell pepper, diced

2 tablespoons crushed walnuts

$\frac{1}{2}$ pint/300 ml/1$\frac{1}{4}$ cups vegetable stock

Parsley, chopped

Lemon juice

Fry the spring onions, garlic and cayenne in the walnut oil until the onions are translucent. Add the fish cubes and red pepper and fry for a further 5 minutes. Add the walnuts and stock and fry for a further 5 minutes.

Serve with chopped parsley and a squeeze of lemon juice.

ROAST VEGETABLES WITH A HOT NUT CRUST

2 tablespoons walnut oil *or* sesame oil

Selection of green vegetables: broccoli, cabbage, celery, chicory, fennel

(continues ...)

1 tablespoon mixed nuts: almonds, walnuts, brazil nuts etc.
1 red chilli, deseeded and finely chopped
1 small slice soft goat's cheese *or* sheep's cheese
Fresh coriander, finely chopped

Pre-heat the oven to 220°C/425°F/gas 7. Heat the oil in a roasting tin in the oven. Place the green vegetables in the tin, rolling them in the oil until evenly coated. Roast until the vegetables are slightly browned and crisped. Whilst the vegetables are roasting crush the nuts in a pestle and mortar or by placing them in a bag and rolling with a bottle, rolling pin or other hard object. Add the chilli to the nuts and sprinkle this mixture over the vegetables for the last few minutes of roasting. When the vegetables are ready, remove them from the oven and place on a plate. Roll the cheese over the cooled roasting tin to coat it with the remaining nut and chilli mix, then place it on the plate with the vegetables and spoon any of the remaining nut mix over the entire dish. Sprinkle with the coriander and serve.

COD AND COLCANNON

Colcannon is a popular Scottish way of serving mashed potato. This is the detox version which leaves out the cream and butter but is just as tasty and far healthier!

2 large potatoes
1 cod steak *or* fillet
1 small leek, finely shredded
1 piece green cabbage (savoy is best), finely shredded
1 clove garlic, crushed
Olive oil
Freshly ground black pepper

Boil the potatoes until soft. Grill the cod on both sides until slightly golden on top. Fry the leek, cabbage and garlic in a little oil until slightly browned. Mash the cooked potatoes together with a tablespoon of olive oil to loosen it. Finally, add the fried vegetables to the potato and roughly blend together. The texture of the dish will be quite rough once it has been mixed with the vegetables. Pile the potato in the centre of a plate and place the grilled cod on top with a sprinkling of black pepper.

SMOKED HADDOCK WITH PINE NUT CRUMBLE

1 tablespoon pine nuts
1 tablespoon chopped fresh coriander
Black pepper
Olive oil
1 fillet smoked haddock (undyed)
Courgettes (zucchini), sliced
1 onion, chopped

Crush together half the pine nuts with all the coriander and some black pepper. Add enough olive oil drop by drop until you have a stiff paste, then add the remaining pine nuts whole. Grill the haddock for 5–6 minutes until cooked through. Fry the courgettes with the onion in more olive oil until just golden. Spread the coriander and pine nut mix on top of the fish and continue to grill until the crumble is browned. Put the courgette and onion mixture on to a heated plate and place the haddock crumble on top. Sprinkle with more black pepper and serve.

SALADE NIÇOISE

1 tuna steak
Olive oil
Mixed herbs, chopped
Lemon juice
New potatoes
Green beans
Lettuce leaves
Black olives
Black pepper
1 clove garlic, chopped
Fresh coriander, chopped
Pine nuts, toasted

Marinate the tuna in some of the olive oil, all the mixed herbs and a little lemon juice for a couple of hours in the fridge, then remove the fish from the marinade and grill until golden. Meanwhile, boil the potatoes until soft and the beans until crunchy. Slice the olives in half and mix them with the cooked potatoes, green beans and lettuce leaves. Pile the mixture on to a warmed plate and place the grilled tuna on top. To make the dressing, blend olive oil, lemon juice, pepper, garlic, coriander and pine nuts and pour over the salad. Serve warm.

ROAST VEGETABLES WITH CHÈVRE BLANC

Olive oil
Selection of vegetables: bell peppers (green and red), courgettes
    (zucchini), chicory, fennel, celery, red onions, kohlrabi
5–6 cloves garlic
Slices of chèvre blanc

Black pepper
Cayenne pepper

Pre-heat the oven to 220°C/42 °F/gas 7. Put 2–3 table-spoons of olive oil into a roasting tin and heat in the oven. Slice the vegetables into bite-size chunks, the rougher the better. Once the oil is really hot put the vegetables and whole garlic cloves in the tin and roll them in the oil to coat evenly. Roast for 10 minutes, then check for burning and roast for a further 5 minutes or so to suit. Once the vegetables are cooked to your liking place slices of the cheese on to them and roast for a further·5 minutes or until the cheese begins to brown. Transfer the contents of the roasting tin to a bowl or plate, sprinkle with black and cayenne pepper and eat whilst hot. The garlic cloves can be eaten whole or squeezed over the vegetables.

Warming Winter Vegetables with Pecorino Romano

Pecorino Romano is a Parmesan-type hard cheese made with sheep's milk.

Olive oil
$\frac{1}{2}$ onion, sliced
3 cloves garlic
Cayenne pepper to taste
Winter vegetables, as many and as varied as you wish
$\frac{1}{2}$ red bell pepper
Fresh ginger, grated
Juice of $\frac{1}{2}$ lemon
7 oz/215 g/1 cup brown rice, cooked
2 oz/60 g Pecorino Romano, grated

Heat the oil and fry the onion, garlic and cayenne for 2 minutes. Chop the vegetables and add them to the pan along with the ginger and lemon juice. Fry for 5 minutes or until the vegetables are softened but not overcooked. Add the rice to the pan and stir-fry together for a further minute. Remove from the heat, stir in some of the Pecorino Romano, and serve with the rest grated over the top of the dish.

PUMPKIN OR SQUASH RISOTTO

3 tablespoons olive oil

4 oz/125 g shallots *or* mild onions, sliced

1 medium pumpkin *or* squash

1½ pints/900 ml/4 cups vegetable stock

1 clove garlic, chopped

15 oz/430 g/2 cups uncooked brown rice

4 oz/125 g Pecorino Romano, grated

Heat the olive oil in a pan and fry the shallots. Scoop the flesh out of the pumpkin (retain the shell and put aside), cut into small cubes and add to the oil together with a cup of stock. Cook for 5 minutes. Add the garlic, the rest of the stock and the rice, and simmer until the rice has absorbed all the fluid. Place the pumpkin shell in a large pan with some boiling water and simmer until the flesh inside the shell has softened. Remove the shell from the pan, dry off the outside and pour away any liquid from the inside. Stir the cheese into the rice mixture, pile it inside the hollow pumpkin and serve with more grated cheese on top.

SAVOURY SAUTÉED POTATOES

New potatoes
3 tablespoons olive oil
1 small onion, sliced
1 small fennel bulb, sliced
1–2 sprigs rosemary
2 cloves garlic
1 small courgette (zucchini), sliced
1 tablespoon lemon juice
Basil, chopped
Fresh coriander, chopped

Boil the new potatoes for 5 minutes. Heat the oil in a pan and fry the onion, fennel and rosemary until the vegetables are soft and lightly browned. Drain the potatoes and add them to the frying pan. Add the garlic and courgette and fry for 10 minutes, until the potatoes are browned. Remove from the heat, add the lemon, basil and coriander, discard the rosemary and serve.

DESSERTS

When you are following the Detox Programme there is little scope for desserts unless they contain fruit. But even these should be avoided as fruit should always be eaten on an empty stomach; if left to sit on top of a full stomach it can cause acidity. Some fruit such as melons contain amino acids that trigger the stomach to release its contents into the intestine just twenty minutes after the food has been eaten. This is fine if the only thing in the stomach is melon, but if it contains other foods as well the result can be a disrupted digestion.

It is best to limit your desserts to yoghurt or cheese for most of the Detox Programme. If you are entertaining there are many recipes to choose from, but just make sure that you keep your own portion small.

APPLE AND SUMMER FRUIT COMPOTE

1 large eating apple
Mixture of cherries, raspberries, strawberries, blueberries etc.
Honey
1 tablespoon sheep's yoghurt
Sesame seeds, toasted

Peel and core the apple, place in a pan with a very little water and gently steam until the fruit is tender. In a separate pan simmer the summer fruits with 1 tablespoon of the honey until they are soft. Place the apple on a plate and pour over the summer fruits. Top with the yoghurt mixed with a teaspoon of the honey, and sprinkle with sesame seeds.

STRAWBERRY SMOOTHIE

10 large strawberries *or* fruit of your choice
2 small pots goat's yoghurt

Put the ingredients into a blender, blend and serve as a shake. Alternatively, if the fruit is frozen to a 'slightly hard' consistency before being placed in the blender the yoghurt will partially freeze and you will have instant ice cream.

GRILLED LEMON AND ALMOND PINEAPPLE

3 rings fresh pineapple
Juice of $\frac{1}{2}$ lemon
1 teaspoon honey
Handful of toasted almonds

Pre-heat the grill on a high setting. Place the pineapple rings on a baking tray, drizzle with the lemon juice and honey and grill on high. Watch continuously, and as soon as the fruit is browned remove it and serve sprinkled with the toasted almonds.

SUMMER FRUIT ICE CREAM

Mixture of raspberries, strawberries, blackcurrants etc.
1 tablespoon honey
1 pot of sheep's yoghurt

Place the fruit and honey in a pan and simmer until the fruit is soft and the honey has melted. Remove from the heat, place in a bowl and leave to cool. When cool, chill in the freezer until nearly frozen. Place the yoghurt in a blender and add the frozen fruit tablespoon by tablespoon, blending after each addition. Serve as soon as the mixture is totally blended – it should have the consistency of soft ice cream.

GREEK STYLE YOGHURT

Goat's *or* sheep's yoghurt
Honey
Pistachio nuts, crushed

Mix all the ingredients together and serve chilled.

ENTERTAINING ON THE DETOX PROGRAMME

Entertaining means providing your guests with pleasant surroundings, wonderful food and great company. Entertaining on the Detox Programme is all of this with the bonus of great, healthy food that will do them good. Let your guests know that you are on the programme, but only once they have arrived. They will be amazed that the sumptuous meal you will have been able to prepare from the food lists can be so good for you. Before you know it you will have all your friends following the programme and asking you for your advice!

As well as you telling them about the detox, they will undoubtedly tell you how good you are looking and how much the programme suits you – this is a really positive aspect of the programme and should be appreciated. You have to put a lot of work and self-control into the programme, and it is right that you should benefit from the results, both inside and out.

On the following pages are some suggested menus from the recipes given above.

Menu 1

Olives to nibble

*

Thai carrot soup

*

Nutty monkfish
Brown rice

*

Grilled lemon and almond pineapple

Menu 2

Sardines with apricots

*

Salmon with watercress
Roast vegetables with chèvre blanc

*

Summer fruit ice cream

Menu 3

Nut salad with Pecorino Romano shavings

*

Cod and colcannon

*

Apple and summer fruit compote

Menu 4

Crunchy red coleslaw with Home-made hummus
*
Salade niçoise
*
Selection of fresh fruit and goat's cheese

Menu 5

Three bean salad with mini rice cakes
*
Smoked haddock with
pine nut crumble
*
Strawberry smoothie

Menu 6

Roast fennel with tuna
*
Pumpkin or squash risotto
*
Greek style yoghurt

It is likely that your guests will be drinking wine. Chilled grape juice with sparkling water is your detox alternative – much more refreshing and it guarantees you a clear head in the morning.

LOGISTICAL PROBLEMS AND SOLUTIONS

No time to have a meal

There are always times during the week when you would skip a meal if you were eating normally. Whilst you are following the Detox Programme you should never miss a meal. This doesn't mean that you must stop everything, whatever the situation, and demand to have food. But it does mean that you should always be prepared and carry some form of light snack that will tide you over until it is more convenient to eat.

Carry a larger than usual handbag when you are detoxing and make sure that you have rice cakes, a pot of hummus or (in cooler weather only) goat's cream cheese, and a small plastic bag of dried fruit and nuts. If you prefer cheese, then a few cubes of Feta in a bag will 'feed' your body. These should take up little space and will keep the hunger satisfied.

Being out with people who are not detoxing

Whatever you do, don't hide the fact that you are detoxing. Talk about the programme – people will be fascinated and ask lots of questions. This means that they will understand your situation, so any decisions about eating out or getting food will automatically include your needs. If you keep the programme quiet it will be harder to 'shoehorn' your requests into their chosen meal plans. There will always be some people who try to make you break the programme as soon as they see the opportunity – 'just one glass of wine won't hurt, surely?' – so letting the whole group know the situation will make it easier to ignore this person.

Talking about the Detox Programme also puts it into perspective for yourself. It is likely that at times you will just be 'doing the programme' as it will have become a part of your everyday life, but it is very important to remind yourself just how effective the programme is and how great you feel. Telling people about it makes you become totally aware of everything that is happening to you and everything that you are doing for yourself.

There's only fast food available

Fast food is great! Baked potatoes are fast food, carrots, cauliflower, rice cakes and hummus are fast food, nuts and seeds are fast food – everything is a fast food if all you have to do is reach into your handbag to get it out. Don't be caught out thinking there is nothing to eat when your friends get a takeaway – have your own takeaway with you all the time.

Feeling hungry while shopping, or meeting friends for coffee

Again, if you have food with you you are likely to be able to satisfy any hunger pangs without leaving the programme. Drinking something will also take away any immediate hunger, so stopping for a cup of herbal tea will give your feet a rest and your body some refreshment.

If you are having tea or coffee with friends, most cafés

offer hot water or herbal teas as an alternative. And if your friends are having cake or biscuits you should ask if the café can supply any fresh fruit. If there is still nothing to eat, just nibble discreetly on some nuts from your handbag.

Eating out and there's nothing detox on the menu

Whether in the most expensive restaurant or the cheapest you can always call the waiter or waitress over and ask if they can put together a salad or a plate of assorted vegetables. Even if a restaurant doesn't show salad anywhere on the menu they will always serve salad garnish on some of their dishes, so asking them to put this together as a main course is easy. Side orders of vegetables are normally served without dressings (check with the waiter or waitress) so these are an obvious option. You can either just order side dishes or ask for these to be made into a main course. Potatoes can be the saving vegetable. If they are baked – great. If they are roasted in vegetable or olive oil – great. And if there is nothing else you can think of then fries cooked in vegetable or seed oil are fine – unsalted!

If you need to eat carbohydrate and there are no potatoes or brown rice available then you may have a small portion of wild or white rice – the less refined the better. But this should only be in extreme cases of hunger!

Chinese or Indian restaurants are likely to cause the biggest problems as these are really the only restaurants that don't serve vegetables unless they are cooked in spicy cream or tomato sauces or with monosodium glutamate. If this is the case then prawns are usually on offer in some form. Any sauce on them should be wiped off with your knife and fork, and if you eat them with plain boiled rice you will not be harming the Detox Programme. Just make sure your next meal contains lots of fresh vegetables to make up the shortfall. In Chinese restaurants you may see 'stir fry' on the menu. Ask if this is without sauce and simply tossed in spices and oil – if so, tuck in!

Restaurants are much more user-friendly than they used to be, and many pride themselves on being able to provide almost anything that you request – put them to the test!

PART 3

Maintenance and Enhancement

6

Diary of a Detox

The easiest way to demonstrate life on the Detox Programme is to take you through the day-to-day diary of someone who has actually done it. This chapter will take you through six days of the programme: two from the start, two from the middle and two towards the end. It shows the different stages you will go through, what to expect to feel and what might happen over the thirty days.

The person who wrote this diary was single, living with a partner and working. As far as the Detox Programme is concerned, being single or married makes no difference. You will either be coaxing your partner to eat the same food or cooking for one – simply adapt the quantities to suit.

Working at home, working at the office, not working or being a mother with children at home and so on are surprisingly interchangeable situations. The adaptations you have to make due to being at work or in a meeting are the same as those you have to make at home surrounded by young children – these are all distractions, and the diary simply demonstrates that with a little forethought you can adapt the programme to suit any lifestyle.

Eating out or entertaining hold the same opportunities

and problems for everyone. You will see that all these demands can be easily coped with whilst you are on the programme.

DAY 1, SUNDAY

Try and be busy on the first day – make sure you have all the right food available and then get going.

The temptation to spend the day with the sole focus of FOOD will be exhausting and very negative.

Got up and turned the shower to cold for approximately five seconds – that will do for Day 1, I think. After drying off I tried out the dry skin brushing, got very hot and my skin was buzzing – felt like I had done a reasonable amount of exercise already.

I decided to clear out the cellar. *After a breakfast of hot water with lemon juice, pears, sheep's yoghurt, sunflower seeds sprinkled on top and some grated ginger*, I set to work.

I also decided to start gently. The forty-seven trips up the stairs out into the garden carrying large boxes of rubbish would count as my twenty minutes of exercise for the day – it took two hours.... I drank about four cups of hot water and found that it actually had quite a lot of flavour.

Lunch was a baked potato, the flesh mixed up with one teaspoon of olive oil to make it creamy and Feta cheese melted on top. All this was served with grated beetroot on top – delicious.

I finished my lunch and set about finally sorting out my holiday photos, something I have been needing to do for a long time. Several trips to the toilet later – just proves that my body is not used to having so much fluid to deal with – I begin to feel like I am actually beginning to flush out. I didn't feel tired or lethargic at any stage during the day and actually feel as if I have got more done than I ever do on a normal Sunday. Perhaps it is symbolic that I chose to 'clean out' and 'sort out' my life on the day that I start to 'clean out' and 'sort out' my body.

Supper at 6.45 of roast vegetables: leeks, onions, fennel, courgettes and broccoli with creamy goat's cheese melted on top and served on a bed of short grain brown rice. I felt like I needed a dessert but ended up with a handful of almonds which had more flavour than I previously remember them having.

When it came to bedtime I still felt quite alert so I massaged both my legs and arms with my normal moisturiser and went to bed.

Had a really good night's sleep.

DAY 2, MONDAY

Woke up really invigorated this morning – didn't want to get out of bed but didn't feel as if I needed more sleep. Went to the gym for half an hour and did ten minutes each on the treadmill, step machine and bike.

Got home, showered and then splashed about in the bath in cold water. Definitely prefer just turning the shower to cold for a few minutes as running the bath was time-consuming. Drank the hot water and dry skin brushed – fitting it all in is OK but will require concentration.

Had the same as yesterday for breakfast. Thought that I was being bad not to use my imagination with all the new fruit to try, but then realised that I have had toast and coffee every morning for the last twenty-two years so having the same whilst on the detox should be no problem.

Had a busy morning in the office and every time I came to drink my hot water it was cold water – just as refreshing. My skin seems to be a tad greasy today. We had a conversation across the office about skin care and no one asked me what I did to keep looking young and beautiful – I suspect it was a tactful way of saying I didn't! I am surprised this has happened so quickly but it is only to be expected if I am cleansing myself.

Lunch was last night's leftover roast vegetables with a salad from the corner sandwich bar – special request to 'hold the tomatoes'. I probably overdid the salad. I thought I might be very hungry so asked for a large green salad and couldn't actually finish it off.

Developed a very mild headache this afternoon so I drank some camomile tea and did some deep breathing. Feels better but not completely gone. This might last a while so I will take a rest as soon as possible.

Needed to drive into town for a meeting. Normally I load up for the two-hour drive with snacks and potato crisps, but had *water and a bag of almonds to nibble on* – felt very virtuous. Drank quite a lot of water but realised that there was nowhere to stop to visit the toilet on the journey so stopped drinking quite as much.

I met up with an old school friend for supper and called ahead to warn her that I was 'detoxing' and would bring my own food if necessary but the menu was: *olives to start as appetisers, black and green. Steamed vegetables: carrot, cauliflower, white and red cabbage all mixed with brown*

rice and sesame and cumin seeds. She had yoghurt and straw-
berries for dessert and I just had the strawberries – it couldn't
have been more detox if she had tried.

Drove home feeling tired but happy that I had
managed to eat out without breaking the programme or
disrupting my hosts' evening. Went to bed with the
headache still mild but not unmanageable – proof that my
body is beginning its clean out.

DAY 14, FRIDAY

I am working in town today and so staying with a friend.
Got up feeling really good. Before I showered and
'brushed' I weighed myself. I have been tempted to do
this every day since I started but decided that I would only
weigh in twice – in the middle and at the end. I know the
programme is not about weight loss, but as I am doing all
this exercise and feel so good and 'lean and clean' it would
be the icing on the cake.

I have lost 3lb – Great! This is good because it is not
too much for two weeks but also accounts for any actual
gain of weight due to fat converting to toned muscle. This
makes me feel even better and so I treat myself for breakfast by having something different from my usual pears
and yoghurt topped with seeds – *I mix together grapes,*
apples and strawberries and mix in some freshly grated root
ginger.

I have begun to see my plate as 'energy food' rather
than just food, and make an effort to get at least four
different-coloured fruits or vegetables for each meal.

Went to work and had a massage treatment at

lunchtime – that was wonderful, but I wish I had booked it for this evening as I really felt like making the most of feeling relaxed. But I had to go straight back to work and then drive home afterwards.

Usually I feel tired driving home this late in the week, but my massage must have been more invigorating than I thought. Came home via the gym and someone said that my skin was positively glowing – and they didn't even know I was on the Detox Programme. It must look as good as it feels.

Supper was delicious. I was cooking for two – and number two had made it quite clear that he was not on the detox! Grilled salmon fillets on a bed of watercress, lightly stir-fried red cabbage and red onions and chargrilled courgettes, all drizzled with olive oil and lime juice and a handful of black olives. We finished with a winter fruits frozen yoghurt (sheep's).

The only thing I crave is a glass of cool white wine, but *apple juice and fizzy water makes a suitable alternative.*

Before going to bed, which is getting later and later as I get more and more energy – it must be difficult to live with a 'detoxer' as you can see their boundless energy whilst you still feel exhausted at the end of every day – I smooth in some massage oil with a little lavender for total relaxation and indulgence.

DAY 15, SATURDAY

Got up quite early today as we have friends coming to stay and I need to do the cleaning and some shopping. Hot lemon water whilst sitting up in bed looking at the post and then a quick shower. Skin brush whilst on the telephone and dressing as I tidied up the bedroom. *Breakfast consisted of a pear and a handful of nuts and seeds in the car on the way to the supermarket.*

Not much lunch to speak of as we walk our friends around town and take them for afternoon tea. *I have herbal tea and a fresh fruit salad* whilst they have coffee and cake. Normally I would find this hard to deal with, but the idea of caffeine seems to fill me with horror and the cake would feel far too stodgy.

We are eating out this evening and I am interested to know how easy it is to do this as so far I have managed to avoid it.

The restaurant came out on top. I had mixed olives to start – the selection of breads with olive oil that the others had did look rather good, but again I didn't miss the bread as I feel it would mess up my clean insides. Roast monkfish on a bed of roast peppers with a hazelnut oil and lime dressing, all with a side salad of rocket in olive oil and lemon – it actually looked much nicer than the risotto that the others chose so I was happily full and satisfied.

I feel really self-righteous at the moment but am keeping it to myself – we had an in-depth discussion over dinner about what food was good and why I couldn't eat certain things. At the end of the day I think if we went back to an original diet, i.e. nothing mixed – which means basically veg, fruit, nuts, beans, pulses, fish, white meat and non-dairy – then I reckon we would all be a lot cleaner and healthier.

I don't feel hungry and I'm looking forward to my weigh-in next Sunday. If I have lost even one more pound that will be absolutely superb!

I didn't massage this evening or this morning as I have awarded myself the day off for doing so well.

DAY 28, WEDNESDAY

Had to get into town early to pick up some printing I have had done, so decided that a trip to the grocer's was in order.

Their ready-prepared green salad looked good and so did their giant raisins and apricots. Got a bag of mixed washed vegetables and toddled on back home.

I now feel that the programme is an integral part of my life. The fact that I haven't even mentioned the self massage and skin brushing etc. this morning means that I am managing to fit them in without even blinking. I have missed them out on a couple of mornings, but when I have realised I have definitely wished I had remembered.

Breakfast was two apples, hundreds of grapes and a handful of jumbo raisins and sultanas whilst I sat at my desk working.

Worked all morning and couldn't believe it when lunchtime arrived. *Lunch was a baked potato, green salad and a big dollop of home-made hummus – this makes the potato really creamy and actually quite wonderful.*

Still at my desk at 6.30, so nipped to the corner shop for *a tin of tuna in veg oil, and had that with the mixed vegetables and some beetroot and Feta. I felt full but not over-full, and I think my tastebuds have been reborn – the flavours are quite brilliant even with something so plain.*

Loads of hot water this evening and I suspect I will have to get up in the night as a result.

Bed and 'drainage massage' before sleep. I have also noted that my sleep is very, very much deeper than it has been in ages. I honestly believe that I now go to sleep and don't wake until the alarm goes off – normally I wake a few times when turning over etc. This is excellent, and I hopt it is one of the lasting results of detox.

DAY 29, THURSDAY

Knew I was going to be very busy today so I started by saying my affirmations to myself several times whilst breathing deeply and slowly before getting out of bed;

> I am successful
> I am healthy
> I feel full of energy
> I am prepared for anything

I have found that saying these makes an immediate difference, and nothing can get me down during the day because 'I am prepared for anything.'

I did my normal morning routine and decided that I will definitely continue to turn the shower to cold but will probably only dry skin brush every few days.

Breakfast has settled down to apples and grapes and I nibble on the seeds throughout the morning in the office. I put a bag of nuts and seeds in my desk at the start of the week and then I can forget having to prepare them every day.

I got out of a meeting very late and all there was to drink was fizzy water so I feel a bit bloated – I definitely find flat or hot water easier to digest.

I didn't have time to exercise at the gym today, so I ran up and down the office stairs four times and walked around the block briskly before I drove home. I miss exercise if I don't get the chance to do at least twenty minutes a day – I generally do forty minutes, which is more than required but feels fine.

I still think I can feel the benefit from my aromatherapy massage on Saturday – I was a bit drowsy immediately afterwards but seem to have even more energy now. My skin feels wonderful – several years younger!

I'm afraid I didn't get time for lunch so I had the last of my rice cakes with some Feta cheese at my desk – the Feta tastes very salty now, so my tastebuds must be completely clean and detecting every flavour I subject them to.

Tomorrow is the last day of the Detox programme for me. I actually think I will miss a lot of the programme, and will probably keep to it during the week and then gradually phase in the things I have missed at weekends. The idea of eating bread or meat isn't very appealing. I will have a glass of wine, but that will be the only thing that I think I have really missed.

As I am working tomorrow evening – my 'last evening' – we planned to eat out tonight to 'celebrate' my achievement: *Red mullet and salmon on a green bean and onion salad, dressed in oil and vinegar, followed by grilled goat's cheese roulade on a bed of roast vegetables and hazelnuts, all washed down with mineral water* – well done me!

Obviously your own days will be very different, but the essence of the eating and detox activities and how you fit them into your day will remain the same. There will be days when you do more towards the Detox Programme than others, but you should definitely include the daily food and activity checklist items as and when required. Missing something out will not mean you should start all over again. It simply means that you will not be getting the greatest benefit from the programme – and as you can see, it really is quite easy to follow.

7

Maintaining the Detox

There are ways to 'come off' the Detox Programme, ways to prolong and maintain the programme, ways to do a 'short detox' programme and mini 'fast' programmes. All these, in combination with the full thirty-day programme, will maintain a permanent state of detox for your body.

The first time you follow the Detox Programme will always be the most challenging, for you will be detoxing the whole of your life to that day – twenty, thirty, forty years or whatever. The second time you undertake the programme you will only be detoxing what has accumulated in the time since your last detox – much easier. Your body will respond much more immediately and the highs of energy that on the first occasion it took between seven and fourteen days to experience will be felt by the end of Week 1. However, it is still very important to detox for the full thirty days each time, as this guarantees thorough cleansing.

'COMING OFF' THE DETOX PROGRAMME

What you do immediately after your first Detox Programme can increase and prolong the effect of detox by many months. But whatever you do after the programme is completed you cannot reverse the good work you have done. Even if you decide to return to burgers and caffeine you will still enjoy the benefits of detox and your body will still thank you for the 'rest' you gave it.

On Day 30 of the Detox Programme you will be looking forward to taking yourself out to dinner or making a meal to reward yourself for all the hard work and self-control you have exercised in the previous month. You should definitely do something to mark your success, but be aware that coming off the programme is as crucial as starting the programme.

Over the last thirty days your body has become used to being nourished with simple foods that it can readily digest and absorb. It has become used to high nutrition. Processed foods, preservatives, additives, chemicals and refined foods have not been part of your diet for a whole month. If you add all these foods back overnight, your body may find it difficult to digest them. This can cause constipation, indigestion, headaches and bloating. If you wish to include in your diet some or all of these 'old' foods, do so slowly and over a period of time to avoid any of these side-effects.

As you start to approach Day 30 you should assess how you feel and think about the things that you wish to reintroduce once the programme has been completed. Make a list of these foods, and also note those that you have really missed. Normally, the things that you have missed will be the types of food to which you may have developed an intolerance before going on the programme. Common examples are white bread, cheese, coffee, wine, sweet cakes, biscuits and red meat.

You should then start to think about how you will *gradually* introduce these into your programme. If you add them one at a time you will be able to monitor how your body responds to them. Then, if there is an adverse reaction you can exclude them or introduce them in much smaller amounts over a longer period of time.

If, for instance, you want to reintroduce bread or refined flour, don't have toast for breakfast, a sandwich for lunch and pasta for supper. It is likely that this kind of overload will make you feel bloated and sluggish. Instead you should have toast on the first day, a salad sandwich on the second and pasta for supper on the third. Check how you feel, and then increase the frequency if all seems well. You may find that a slice of breakfast toast is enough to satisfy your bread requirements, so try to remember how much good you have done for your body and how reducing items like refined flours will prolong the effects of the detox.

It is also likely that rich or very creamy foods will upset your stomach. Treat these with care. Again, excluding these foods or only eating them very occasionally will prolong the effects of your detox.

Don't be surprised if there are some foods that you would have previously considered as regular staples in your diet, but which you now find difficult to eat. Your taste may well have changed and their flavour is no longer acceptable. These foods are generally meat, dairy foods and those with strong or salty flavours. Over a period of time they will become acceptable to you again if you eat them in small amounts. But again this may be a great opportunity to cut these foods out permanently, especially if they are processed or contain a lot of additives.

MAINTAINING THE DETOX PROGRAMME

As well as watching the sorts of foods you reintroduce when you have completed the thirty days, you should also note the foods from the Detox Programme that you want to keep as a staple part of your new healthier diet. If you wish to 'stop' the programme and return to how you were eating previously, there are still parts of the programme that you can continue with without restricting your choices. Combining your eating habits in this way will supplement any areas of deficiency. By keeping some of the regular supplements from the detox in your diet, you will be maintaining your detox.

The easiest parts of the Detox Programme to stick with when you have finished are those that take very little time and can be done without really having to think about them.

Drink a cup of hot water and lemon juice first thing every morning

Whether you are on the Detox Programme or not, starting the day with hot water and lemon is very refreshing, cleansing for your liver and invigorating. It is just as easy to add lemon juice as it is to put a teaspoon of coffee or a teabag in your mug – and much better for you.

During the day drink 3 pints (1.7 litres) of water

Once you have got into the habit of drinking lots of water during the Detox Programme it is much easier to carry on than to stop. Your body will have become used to the extra fluids, and reducing the quantity will make you thirsty. There is no good reason to stop the water intake – so don't!

Take two liver tonics a day

A small snack of a handful of black grapes, plus a cup of fennel tea, every day should be easy enough to maintain, and if you remind yourself of the benefits it becomes even easier.

Take two kidney tonics a day

Adding a teaspoon of honey to your lemon juice and taking a cranberry supplement at breakfast takes no time, and the benefits are continually invigorated kidneys.

Eat three meals every day

Three meals a day is very important, even if they are non-detox meals. Leaving long gaps in between meals or skipping meals will disrupt the body's delicate metabolism and push it into starvation mode. Eating four to six small meals a day is infinitely preferable to having two or three meals with large gaps in between.

The effects

Continuing with the aspects of the programme listed above will:

• Act as a tonic to your liver and kidneys

- Cleanse your palate and intestines

- Flush out any toxins you consume

- Keep the pH balance in your body regulated

- Maintain a good metabolic rate

Coupled with your new detoxed body, these habits will maintain a constant cleansing process. They should take no more than five minutes out of your day.

FASTING, MINI FASTS AND MINI MINI FASTS

Fasting has been popular for many hundreds of years and claims to be a way of totally cleansing your insides. It means eating nothing and drinking only water. Fasting allows the body to cleanse itself of waste and empty the systems of all residual foods. The clearer the path, the more efficiently the body can absorb and use all nutritional foods. Fasting also facilitates the release of hormones that stimulate the immune system.

Various different lengths of fast can be undertaken, but if you wish to complete a fast of three days or more it must always be done under the supervision of your GP/doctor. The side-effects of long-term fasting – without correct supervision and instruction – can do more harm than good. Literally starving your body for more than twenty-four hours will lead to feelings of weakness, nausea and dizziness, muscle fatigue and dehydration. If you try to operate normally – going to work, looking after the family and so on – you are likely to suffer major lapses in concentration and extreme fatigue. Any existing health conditions will be exacerbated by lack of nourishment.

There are other forms of fasting that are less severe and, in my view, much more effective. Restricting your diet to certain types of cleansing foods for between twenty-four and forty-eight hours, but no longer, can help to maintain and/or boost the Detox Programme.

Once you have completed the programme you may find times when you think you have eaten too many processed foods, or have had to eat out a lot and don't feel as if you have been very kind to your body. At times like these you can try a mini fast. You can also think about trying a mini mini fast more regularly – perhaps once a week on an evening when you are not going out.

If you fast after you have detoxed it will bring positive results immediately. Each time you fast you are just flushing out the small build-up of toxins and waste. Fasting regularly after detox will maintain the detox at its fullest potential.

Don't just decide to fast and then starve yourself for the next few days. Fasting must be thought through, and preparation is essential if you are to get the best results.

How to fast

Check that you fulfil the necessary health requirements, as with the Detox Programme:

- You are not pregnant

- You are not breastfeeding

- You do not suffer from any illness or heart condition
- You are not diabetic
- You are not taking prescribed drugs
- You have no doubts about your own personal health

Decide when you want to fast and for how long – a mini fast is eighteen hours and a mini mini fast fourteen hours.

As with the detox plan, you must start and finish gradually. Leading up to the fast you should cut out caffeine, red meat, processed foods and alcohol. The last three meals before your fast should all be from the Detox Programme.

Throughout the fast you should:

- Drink plenty of hot water, lemon juice and honey
- Take Vitamin C supplements every four hours, or a timed release supplement
- Drink at least 3 pints (1.7 litres) of fluid in the form of water, herbal teas, or apple, grape or lemon juice
- Have some black grapes to nibble on in case your hunger becomes unbearable

Once you have finished your fast you should eat only foods from the Detox Programme for a day, and then slowly introduce normal foods in the same way you would when finishing the Detox Programme.

The mini fast

This fast can be done once a month and will give your body the 'time out' it needs to cleanse internally. The mini fast takes place overnight, so you are only aware of fasting for around ten hours. It lasts from 6 p.m. until 3 p.m. the following day. Having eaten detox foods during the day you should:

- At 6 p.m. eat a light vegetarian meal, ideally from the Detox Programme

- Eat nothing until 3 p.m. the following day, but make sure you drink plenty of herbal teas, juices or water during the early evening and following day

- At 3 p.m. have a light snack of fruit, salad and brown rice

- At 6 p.m. have another meal of fresh fruit and vegetables

The mini mini fast

This fast should be done once a week and can probably be done without really noticing you are on a fast! As with the mini fast, you are actually asleep for most of the time so it feels like a short four- or five-hour fast. But even fasting for such a short time gives your body time to process and cleanse itself.

Getting into the habit of eating your final meal of the day as early as possible will give your body a better chance to digest the foods correctly. Detox or not, the benefits of proper digestion should not be underestimated. The mini mini fast takes place from 6 p.m. to 8 a.m. the following day. Having eaten detox foods during the day you should:

- At 6 p.m. eat a light vegetarian meal, ideally from the Detox Programme

- Eat nothing until 8 a.m. the following day, but make sure you drink plenty of herbal teas, juices or water during the early evening

- At 8 a.m. have a light breakfast of hot water and lemon juice, fruit, goat's or sheep's yoghurt and seeds

- At lunchtime have another meal of fresh fruit and vegetables

You have now completed a fully functional fast with all the benefits and few 'hunger pains'. NB: This fast is most effective if you have already completed the thirty-day detox.

8

Second Time Around: the Short Detox

The Detox Programme is spread over thirty days to ensure that your body has time to adapt and then become used to a new, more healthy way of operating. The gradual changes become permanent if you take them slowly. Reports say that if you want to give something up you should exclude it from your diet for between one and three months, after which you stop craving it.

However, there may be times when you want to follow the Detox Programme but you don't have thirty days available, or you have already completed the full programme and would like to do a shortened version once in a while. This is where the Short Detox Programme can be followed. It is slightly more severe, but as you are trying to pack thirty days into ten more immediate changes are required. The ten-day programme is ideally suited to those who have already completed the full programme, as the work required by your internal organs (liver, kidneys, lymph etc.) will be reduced if you have already detoxed in the past year or so. Indeed, you are not recommended to follow the short programme unless you have completed the full one, or it could be too much of a shock for your body.

If you follow the ten-day plan you will find that the

reactions you got in the thirty-day pr... gerated: headaches may be stronger tiredness will be more immediate but wi time, energy levels will hit a high very skin will look dull for a couple of days radiant. The ten-day detox is a comple body, and if you are prepared for some quite remarkable changes very rapidly it is a great experience.

All the principles and allowable foods are the same as in the thirty-day programme. The difference is simply the period of time and the way you schedule and prepare your food. The differences from the thirty-day programme are shown in *italics*.

When you start the detox programme, from Day 1 to Day 10 you must:

- Cold shower every morning

- Do dry skin brushing every morning *and every evening*

- Self massage every morning *and every evening*

- Drink a cup of hot water, *honey* and lemon juice first thing every morning

- During the day drink 3 pints (1.75 litres) of water

- Take two liver tonics as described

- Take two kidney tonics as described

- Take kelp supplements every day

- Take multivitamin supplements *every day*

- Eat three meals every day

rice every day, preferably short grain brown rice

- Have three portions of *raw vegetables every day*

- Have three portions of fruit every day. *NB: You must not eat fruit for any meal other than breakfast*

- Have a selection of salad, non-dairy yoghurt or cheese, pulses, nuts and herbs every day

- Take *forty minutes' exercise every day*

- Have *fifteen minutes' relaxation every day*

- Have *ten minutes of quality breathing every day*

- Say five affirmations and five visualisations ten times each every day

- Smile or laugh heartily every day

- *Exfoliate every day*

- Have an Epsom salts bath every three days

- Have four aromatherapy, massage or reflexology treatments during the ten days

COLD SHOWER EVERY MORNING

When bathing or showering in the mornings, simply turn the shower to cold just before you are ready to finish and let the water run over your entire body for one minute. Alternatively, when you have finished your bath you can turn on the cold tap as the bathwater is draining away, cup your hands under the water and splash it all over your body.

DRY SKIN BRUSHING

1. Find a natural bristle brush or loofah, or a dry flannel or mitt. The bristles or flannel etc. should be firm but not hard, since you will be brushing your skin quite vigorously all over your body – the skin on your stomach is softer than on your shins or forearms. Do not wet or moisturise the skin, as they may cause dragging.

2. Undress to your underwear or preferably take all your clothes off. Stand or sit in a position that gives you access to all parts of the body – the edge of the bed with your feet on pillows is quite good, or else try sitting on the edge of the bath with one foot up on the toilet seat if it is close enough.

3. Start at the feet and systematically work up towards the top of your body. All strokes should be towards the heart – the heart is a wonderful machine for pumping blood down and throughout the body, but both blood and lymph need extra help to work against gravity to return through the system. If you brush away from the heart it may cause faintness or disrupt the normal flow. Each stroke should be long and firm. Place the brush or mitt on your ankle and firmly brush up to your knee. Repeat until you have covered the entire calf and shin several times. When you have completed the lower leg move up to your knee. The next strokes should run from your knee to the top of your thigh and over your buttocks.

4. Then brush both arms, from the wrist to the shoulder.

The neck and shoulder area should be treated more gently as the flesh here is very delicate. Work from the top of your arm, up and over your shoulder, and gently up your neck to the base of your skull.

5. When brushing your stomach, use gentle circular strokes in a clockwise direction. This will follow the flow in your intestines and not disrupt any bowel functions.

6. You must only brush your face with a soft facial brush or flannel, as the skin here is very delicate and can be damaged if the brush is too hard.

The whole process should only take three or four minutes, and you should feel invigorated when you have finished. Your skin will tingle and you should feel quite warm, as you will have stimulated and increased your circulation. You will soon notice a difference in your skin: it feels smoother, with a softer texture, and the dry patches will all have disappeared. Just spend a little time each day and you will be pleasantly surprised.

SELF MASSAGE

Most normal massage strokes can be converted to be used for self massage. As long as you observe the general rules of massage, even 'made up' strokes will be perfectly acceptable and effective.

• As with dry skin brushing, all massage strokes should be towards the heart. Pushing the blood around the system should be done in conjunction with the circulation and not against it.

- All strokes should be using either the flat hand (fingers together, palms down) or the ends of the fingers (bunched together, no fingernails)

- All massage strokes should start lightly and slowly build to a firmer, more rapid pace.

- The flesh should be warm and relaxed before any deeper strokes can be used. Working deeply on cold, tense flesh will feel unpleasant and cause bruising.

- Massage should never be painful or sore, but massage that is too light is little better than a comforting stroke.

- You should be relaxed when carrying out self massage, as you need to work in some awkward positions and don't want to cause any twists or injuries.

Where possible, you should make sure the room you are in is warm and quiet, perhaps with some relaxing or calming music. If the room is cold it is likely that you are not totally relaxed, which will not result in the best massage.

Use a massage oil, favourite cream or body lotion and apply just enough to let your hands work over the flesh firmly. If you use too much you will just slip over the skin, and if you use too little you may pull or 'burn' the skin. Reapply as necessary, and if you apply too much just wipe the excess on another part of the body until you need it later.

HOT LEMON AND HONEY WATER

The biggest organ of detox is the liver, so starting the day with a squeeze of fresh lemon juice in a cup of hot water will not only refresh and revitalise you but will also clean your palate and 'jump start' your liver. Cider vinegar can be substituted, but may be a little sharp for most palates. Adding honey makes the drink even more cleansing for the bowel.

WATER

You must drink 3 pints (1.7 litres) of water every day. Around 80 per cent of our bodies consist of water and we need to keep that level stable. In hot weather or when you are taking exercise you should increase this amount to cover the deficit. Water replenishes, cleanses, rejuvenates and restores, and is probably the most important single item in the Detox Programme.

LIVER TONICS

You must have the following two liver tonics every day:

- A clove of fresh garlic (in food, not on its own) or an odourless garlic tablet (a high dose tablet is best)

- A large glass of pure carrot and beetroot juice. You can make this yourself or buy fresh juices from health food shops

KIDNEY TONICS

You must have the following two kidney tonics every day:

- A teaspoon of honey in a cup of hot water, sipped slowly

- A medium glass of cranberry juice or a cranberry tablet supplement

SUPPLEMENTS

You must have the following supplements each day:

- Kelp tablets: kelp is a good source of iodine, which keeps the metabolic rate balanced

- Multivitamin: vitamin supplements will ensure that any problems or shortfalls in the early stages of the programme will not leave your body short of essential nutrients. You must take these supplements every day of the intensive ten-day detox.

THREE MEALS A DAY

You must have at least three meals per day. Breakfast should be before 9 a.m., lunch before 2 p.m. and your evening meal before 7 p.m. Even better is to have 4–6 smaller meals, which avoids large spans of time without eating and thus enables your body to cleanse and detox itself without any blood-sugar lows.

BROWN RICE

You must have a large portion of brown rice every day. It acts as a sponge that travels through the gut collecting all the silt and waste, and then flushes it out. During the ten-day intensive detox you must make sure that your body is absorbing and expelling the waste as efficiently as possible.

OTHER FOOD

All the other permitted foods are fruit, raw vegetables, salads, non-dairy milk, yoghurt and cheese, pulses, herbs and nuts, and are exactly the same as in the lists in Chapter 4. In order to get a healthy spread of necessary nutrients you must have some of each of these foods every day. If you miss out a food category you may begin to feel lethargic.

EXERCISE

You should do at least forty minutes' exercise every day during the ten-day Detox Programme. Not only will this help to keep you fit and toned, but it will also ensure that your metabolic rate does not decrease or your circulation become sluggish.

BREATHING

You must have ten minutes of quality breathing every day.

1. Sit comfortably or lie down, supporting your lower back if necessary.

2. Place your hands on your stomach area with your fingertips just touching.

3. Start to breathe in through your nose very slowly to a count of four. As you inhale you should feel your stomach expand and your fingertips separate.

4. Hold the breath for four and exhale slowly through your mouth to a count of eight.

5. Repeat several times as required.

It will feel strange at first as you are not used to using your muscles to expand your stomach in this way, but over a period of just a few minutes this will become more natural.

Continue this exercise for at least ten inward breaths and you should feel much more relaxed and 'centred'. Eventually you will not need to use your fingers to check that your stomach is expanding rather than your chest, and soon you will be able to carry out the exercise whilst you are going about your normal day-to-day business (not the lying down, but the controlled breathing!). If you ever have difficulty in dropping off to sleep, this is a far more effective way than the traditional 'counting sheep'. The chances are that you won't make it to ten, but will probably be asleep by six.

AFFIRMATIONS AND VISUALISATIONS

You must say five affirmations and do five visualisations ten times each every day. These are ways to think and see yourself reaching your goals and achieving your own success in a personal way. When you have been doing them for a while you will notice subtle changes and your friends and colleagues will keep saying how much more positive and 'up' you seem. See pp.74–77 for more information on these techniques.

RELAXATION

You must have fifteen minutes of total relaxation every day:

1. Find a quiet room, make sure you are warm and choose some melodic, peaceful music.

2. Lie down on the floor or sit comfortably in a chair.

3. Close your eyes and start to breathe deeply as described in the breathing exercise on p.155.

4. After breathing correctly for a couple of minutes you should find that your breathing has slowed down and you feel very natural.

5. When you inhale, imagine that the air you are breathing is warm and golden and is bathing your body in warm, golden, restful and positive light.

6. Now start to consider how your body is feeling. As you inhale start thinking about the feet and ankle area of your body. Are they tense? If so, relax them.

7. As you exhale picture the air you breathe out to be the old stagnant air and the air you breathe in is the new, fresh air.

8. Think of your calves and knees. Picture the warm air travelling through any tense muscles, bathing them in light. Exhale the stale air.

9. Picture your knee joints and your upper leg area. Breathe deeply and relax.

10. Feel the air being breathed into the groin area, relaxing the tension and soothing the pelvis. Breathe out the bad air.

11. See the golden light swirling around your stomach and abdomen, cleansing and uplifting your centre of emotion and spirit.

12. Watch the light thread its way between each rib, filling your lungs and chest cavity with warm expanding air.

13. Watch each finger fill with golden light which spreads through your fingers and lower arms.

14. Breathe in the energy into your shoulders and base of your neck. Feel your neck relax and melt into the floor or back of the chair and up into the base of your skull.

15. The light may now travel into the root of each hair follicle, making your scalp feel invigorated and tingling.

16. Each time you exhale you are breathing out waste. Each time you breathe in you are breathing in new life.

17. When you have renewed the life inside your body, look to see where the source of your new breath and new light is coming from.

18. With your eyes still closed, look above you and see the beam of light coming down towards your body. See it feeding into your abdomen. You are connected to this light and you can take as much as you wish.

19. Breathe deeply and inhale all you need.

20. When you are ready you can start to think about bringing your consciousness back into your own body and into the room you are in.

21. Open your eyes slowly. If you are lying on the floor or bed, roll over on to your side and wait a few moments before pushing yourself up to first a sitting and then a standing position.

22. You should now feel totally relaxed and invigorated – well done!

EXFOLIATION

You must exfoliate every day. Run a bath and put a few drops of your favourite bath oil or foam into the water. Get in and relax! Allow at least ten minutes before you start to exfoliate, which will give you time to relax and your skin time to soften.

You now have two options. For the first, get out of the bath, making sure the bathroom is still nice and warm, and gently rub your exfoliating cream or home-made exfoliant (see p.82) in firm circles, large and small, all over your body. Pay special attention to areas of hard skin such as heels, knees and elbows, and rub as hard as you find comfortable. The whole process should take about three to four minutes. When you have completed the 'rub' get back into the bath and carry on the circular rubbing until all the cream has been washed off into the bathwater. Get out of the bath and then rub yourself dry with a towel (not one that has been rinsed in fabric conditioner, which increases its absorbency and will carry on the exfoliating process as you are drying yourself). Once dry, apply a good moisturiser or body oil all over your body and stay warm, perhaps by going to bed.

Your second option is to stay in the bath and lift each limb above the surface of the water, then exfoliate as described above, in firm circles, large and small. As you finish each limb lower it back into the water and continue to work the flesh until all the cream has been washed away. The only area that may get neglected using this method is the buttocks, but you can do them by kneeling up in the bath. Towel dry as above, then moisturise and keep warm.

EPSOM SALTS BATHS

You must take an Epsom salts bath every three days. Run a deep bath warm enough to sit in for ten or fifteen minutes without going cold. Pour abour 2lb (1kg) of Epsom salts (available from chemists or health food stores) into the bath and stir until it has all dissolved. Get into the bath and have ready a glove or massage mitt.

Sit in the bath for at least five minutes before you start to massage your body. Start massaging with slow, gentle strokes, and as you get used to it make the strokes more vigorous. You may get very warm quite quickly. If this happens slow down your massage and just let the Epsom salts work on you as you relax.

When you get out of the bath you should pat yourself dry and then wrap up warmly for the next hour or so. Ideally the bath should be taken in the evening just before you go to bed, which will keep you warm for many hours. Alternatively you can take your bath during the day, then wrap up in a quilt or blanket and sit and watch an old movie!

ADDITIONAL TREATMENTS

During the ten days you must have four aromatherapy, massage or reflexology treatments (see Chapter 9).

9

Ways to Enhance the Detox Programme

There are several ways in which you can enhance the Detox Programme, speed up the process, increase your awareness of your body and make the Detox Programme positively luxurious. If you choose not to do any of the treatments mentioned in this section you will not harm the detox process, but you will not be giving your body the ultimate detox environment. They are most definitely 'enhancements' and not just 'extras'. As mentioned before, detox is a combination of elements designed to provide the optimum conditions for the body to cleanse itself in every aspect, physical, emotional and mental. Any of the following treatments can also be used for stress reduction and stress management.

You have already made a decision to implement some major, exciting and positive changes in your life when you undertake the Detox Programme. So why not make it the most enjoyable experience you can through carrying out the equally beneficial but quite luxurious enhancements – you do deserve them.

AROMATHERAPY

Many people believe that aromatherapy is simply a form of nice-smelling massage. But aromatherapy is much more than this, and warrants a book of its own. However, just looking at its origins and effects will give some indication of how it can become part of your everyday life and more specifically part of your detox.

The plant-extracted essential oils used in aromatherapy are absorbed into our bodies via the skin or through inhalation. Initial doubt as to whether substances can be absorbed through the skin has been eliminated by the introduction of 'patches' for many conditions by the medical industry. Once in the bloodstream the molecules travel to the brain and trigger the necessary functions relevant to the specific oil used. If we inhale the essential oil fragrance, the molecules travel inside the nostrils and reach the brain through the thin membranes in the nasal passage and the olfactory system. Inhaling the oils is the quickest way to benefit from them (sniffing drugs has always been the quickest way to experience the effects).

The use of aromatherapy oils is recorded as early as 3000 BC. The Egyptians used oils for medical and cosmetic purposes as well as for embalming. The Greeks and Romans used them in medical practice, and medieval documents contain many references to herbal and scented oils. During the eighteenth and nineteenth centuries substances such as morphine, caffeine and quinine were recorded as ingredients obtained from medicinal plants, and even in the present day we still use plant extracts such as lavender and peppermint in common drugs. Indeed, some of the most powerful drugs available today are derived from plants: heroin, cannabis and digitalis, to name but a few.

Aromatherapy oils are therefore not to be regarded lightly – they can be dangerous if used incorrectly or in the wrong amounts. They are not just pleasant-smelling substances but strong, effective drugs that can have both subtle and sweeping effects on the body, mind and emotions. Many of the oils should only be used by a qualified aromatherapist, and none should be used without reference to a book or leaflet on the subject. You should not just choose an oil because you like the smell – it may have side-effects or contra-indications that can be harmful or downright dangerous.

Essential oils should never be used if you believe you are pregnant or if you are trying to become pregnant, unless otherwise prescribed by a trained aromatherapist. Nor should essential oils ever be taken internally.

Treatment or home use

During an aromatherapy massage treatment the client lies on a massage couch, either naked or in their underwear, covered in towels or blankets to keep warm. The room should be warm and the practitioner should have a calm, relaxing approach. The treatment will usually last about an hour. You may feel drowsy after the session, but a glass of water will soon remedy this.

Alternatively you can use aromatherapy in your own home as the benefit of the oils is not restricted to use in massage, and the appropriate oil can be used for almost every condition or situation. For the purpose of this book, however, I shall concentrate on those oils that are particularly useful during detox because they have cleansing and supportive properties.

Oils for detox

There are a huge number of essential oils available today. The following list includes oils that are specific to detox. If you are aware of any other oils that you would like to use or are currently using other oils, these may be combined in any of the methods prescribed.

Juniper

An astringent, antiseptic and detoxifying oil, juniper is often used as a tonic as it can help to speed up a sluggish circulation and increase elimination. Juniper is a diuretic – it will relieve the retention of urine – and therefore increases the expulsion of toxins and waste. It speeds up the metabolic rate, which in turn increases the detox rate. As a 'cleansing' oil it works both on a physical and an emotional level – it detoxes both mind and body.

Fennel

A great oil for the digestion, fennel strengthens peristalsis – the contraction of the intestinal muscles. Fennel is also a diuretic and so prevents water retention. It works as an antiseptic in the urinary tract and kidneys, dealing with any germs and maintaining a favourable environment during detox. Finally, it is a general tonic and helps to increase circulation and remove waste and toxins.

Rosemary

One of the best all-round essential oils, rosemary is a great balancer of moods and physical manifestations. It has a wonderful stimulating effect on the central nervous system and the rest of the body, and is one of the best oils to use as a natural pick-me-up. Rosemary is a tonic for the heart, skin, kidneys, spleen and blood; it also stimulates the circulation and boosts low blood pressure. However, it should not be used by people who have epilepsy.

Lemon grass

A cleansing, refreshing, spicy oil, lemon grass stimulates the digestion and eases any nervous stomach conditions. It promotes the removal of toxins from the body and is antiseptic and bactericidal.

Peppermint

Used as a remedy for digestive problems, peppermint helps the stomach, liver and intestines. It will ease any strain placed on the intestines and stomach during detox, and will decrease swelling and any bloating. Peppermint can also be used to stimulate the mind! Cooling and relaxing, it is often used in stomach pills and in cooling leg or foot balms.

Pine

Best used for inhalations or burning as it is a very strong oil, pine is refreshing, uplifting and stimulating. It has a stimulating effect on the circulation and helps to remove any phlegm or mucous conditions caused by detoxing.

Basil

Stimulating to the brain and uplifting to the mind, basil is used for stomach complaints and can help the digestive system during detox. It boosts confidence and the circulation, and increases low energy. However, it is very potent and so should be used sparingly.

Massage

Essential oils should never be applied directly to the skin without first being diluted. This is because they are highly concentrated and can cause irritation or burning in their undiluted state (more than a ton of petals can be required to provide just 2ml of essential oil).

They should be diluted in what are known as carrier oils or base oils – the vegetable or seed oils that we use every day in our kitchens. This may seem a bit crude, but such oils are totally natural and can therefore be absorbed by the skin and act as a moisturiser. Olive, sunflower, safflower, grapeseed, nut and sesame oils are all readily available; macadamia, sweet almond, jojoba and avocado oils are slightly more exotic but can be found in health food stores and some more enlightened chemists.

The ratio of any home-made blend of massage oils should be no more than eight drops of essential oil to every 20ml of carrier or base oil. You should only blend sufficient oils for immediate use – essential oils are a natural preservative, but if stored incorrectly the blend can become stale or rancid.

Take a plastic bottle or bowl and pour in 20ml of base oil. Add your desired essential oil drop by drop and stop when the blend has a sufficiently strong fragrance for your taste – some oils are stronger than others and you may only need two or three drops. Remember, eight drops is the maximum – it is always better to have less essential oil than more, because using too much can sometimes cause headaches.

Use the blend as you would in a normal massage, or follow the self massage sequence in Chapter 4. When the massage is complete try to keep the oil on your skin for at least an hour, which will allow the essential oil to continue being absorbed. If you need to dress after a massage, wipe off any excess oil first because it may colour or stain your clothing.

Bathing

As with massage, essential oils should never be used before being diluted in base or carrier oils (see above) or a dispersant. The two most readily available dispersants in the average household are milk or high-volume alcohol (vodka is best, as it has no fragrance and no sugar content). These products will break down the essential oil into much smaller droplets, which will make it spread more evenly in the water and be less likely to irritate your skin.

Diluting your essential oil with a base or carrier oil will make your bath more oily. This is great when you can massage the residue of oil into your skin after the bath, but if you are bathing first thing in the morning or if you need to get dressed immediately afterwards a dispersant is more practical, since it will immediately be absorbed into the skin without leaving any greasy residue.

When bathing in oils you should not use soap, which

would destroy their effect. Choose a time when you do not need to wash, such as just before bed or after you have taken a quick shower. Run a bath that is hot enough to stay warm for fifteen or twenty minutes but not too hot to be uncomfortable to sit in.

Decide whether to use a carrier oil or a dispersant. In either case you only need a tablespoon of it. Add between two and four drops of essential oil. When the bath is full, let the water go calm and then sprinkle the tablespoon of blended oil over the surface.

Close all the windows so that none of the steam escapes. You might also want to light some candles to create a really relaxing, sensuous experience. Slowly get into the bath, then concentrate on breathing slowly and deeply, inhaling all the vapour of the oil. Allow your skin to soak and absorb all the oils. You should be able to relax totally and unwind. Try to detox your mind!

When you have finished your bath get out slowly. If you have used a carrier oil, try to smooth all the oil from the surface of the water over your skin. Pat yourself dry, letting as much oil as possible stay on your skin as a natural moisturiser and allowing any residual oil to continue to be absorbed. If you have used a dispersant, there will still be a small amount of oil to massage into your skin. If you need to dress after your bath you should be able to let the oil be absorbed as you would a body cream.

Ideally you should now relax or go straight to bed.

Inhalation

Using essential oils for inhalation is an excellent way to benefit from them immediately without having to remove any clothing. If you breathe in the vapour from the oils they will enter the olfactory system instantly, so you must take care with the amounts used.

First boil some water and pour it into a large bowl. Add two or three drops of your chosen oil – no dispersants or carriers are required as the oil does not come into direct contact with the skin – and lower your head, covered with a towel or sheet, over the bowl. Inhale slowly through your nose and out through your mouth. You can lower your face closer to the water as you become used to the vapour. Inhaling is an excellent method of dealing with colds and coughs as the effects are immediate and the relief is very welcome. Inhale for about five minutes or until you have had enough, then uncover your head and breathe the cool air.

You can also inhale oils by placing two or three drops on an old handkerchief (the oils may stain) and holding it near your nose or mouth. Don't put the hankie directly on the skin as the oils may irritate it.

Compresses

Sometimes nothing more than a hot water bottle is required to relieve discomfort or pain. Using a compress is the aromatherapy equivalent.

Fill a large bowl with hand-hot water, add a couple of drops of your chosen essential oil and soak a large piece of cotton cloth in it for a couple of minutes. Wring out the cloth and fold it into a compress large enough to cover the area of discomfort. Put two further drops of your oil directly on to the compress (it will spread and dilute into the soaked cotton), then hold the compress on the painful place. Use the compress until it cools down, and if you wish you can repeat the process.

The compress method is ideal for period pains, fever, headaches and so on, as the oil can be applied directly in a soothing, relaxing way. You can of course use the compress for any condition or any reason. If you get a brief chance to sit down and relax during your busy day, a nice lavender and ylang ylang compress (both are oils for relaxation and rejuvenation) would make your five minutes even more relaxing!

Burners

An oil burner is an excellent way of getting essential oils into the atmosphere so that you can benefit from their therapeutic qualities as you go about your everyday business. NB: Oils should not be used when there are children under five in the room or house.

The choice of burner is quite important as there are lots that look quite wonderful but are not too practical. You need one with a bowl big enough to contain 120ml of water (the equivalent of a small cup). If the bowl holds much more than this it will take too long to heat the water, and if it is much smaller it will have burnt dry, giving a rancid smell, before the candle has gone out.

You need to fill the burner with water, light the candle below and then put four or five drops of your chosen oil on the surface of the water. You are unlikely to find you have used too much oil in a burner as the vapour will be distributed throughout the building, but if you start to develop a mild headache simply add more water or blow out the candle.

The alternative is to use dry burners – the terracotta rings that go on light bulbs, or the electrically heated porcelain plates. You put a few drops of your chosen oil on the heated surface, and the heat creates the vapour. They can be controlled by either turning off the power or removing the terracotta burner.

MASSAGE

Alongside aromatherapy, massage is one of the oldest-known forms of complementary therapy. As with aromatherapy, massage can be done in isolation (for instance face massage or foot massage) or in total (a massage incorporating every part of the body including the stomach and abdomen).

Traditional massage works by increasing the circulation, which in turn helps the efficient flow of lymph. This has a positive effect on the immune system and keeps the body balanced and healthy. During the Detox Programme any therapy that enhances these functions should be encouraged and enjoyed as much as possible. Muscle conditions such as soreness, spasm and tension are all helped with massage, as the increased blood flow and manipulation techniques help to stretch and tone. There are many other side-effects of these benefits – better skin tone, relaxed mind, lowered heart rate and so on.

We tend to think of massage as 'Swedish' or 'therapeutic' or 'holistic'. There is not much difference between these, as all massage strokes derive from three original 'Swedish' named techniques.

- *Effleurage*: flat hands push flesh from the lower body up towards the head and back down the body. This technique is used to warm the muscles and flesh and to increase the circulation prior to deeper work.

- *Pettrissage*: kneading, wringing and pulling the muscles so that the flesh and muscles are worked against each other or the flesh is pressed against the bone to cause deeper friction. This technique is used to tone the muscles and flesh and to work through any tension or spasm.

- *Tapotement*: quick, invigorating strokes such as hacking (the side of the hand is used to 'chop' the flesh); cupping (cupped hands are placed in rapid succession on the flesh to 'draw' the blood to the surface); and pummelling (hands clenched in fist shapes and placed flesh down in rapid succession on the flesh to cause a deeper impression on the muscles and so increase circulation).

There are many other types of massage – remedial, sports, tai, Indian head and so on. All of these are very valuable, but for the detox process the traditional aromatherapy and massage techniques are the best.

Massage practitioners will use either oils such as the base or carrier oils described for aromatherapy, or a blend of carrier oils and some basic essential oils. During a massage the client lies on a couch, either naked or in underwear, covered in towels or a blanket to keep warm. The room should be warm and peaceful. All massage strokes should be carried out towards the heart as this helps complete the passage of blood throughout the body and increases the circulation of both blood and lymph.

Initial strokes should be relaxing, warming and smooth and should not cause any pain – there may be discomfort, but actual pain is incorrect. Strokes should work in time with your breathing and be of a regular pace. As the treatment progresses and the muscles get warmed the strokes can become more vigorous and more intrusive as the practitioner 'milks' the muscles of any toxins and drains the body of any wastes. Once an area has been warmed, very deep, specific work can be carried out which may feel uncomfortable but will help to sort out deep-seated problems or tense muscle conditions.

Whatever the reason for your massage, it should give an overall feeling of relaxation and wellbeing if carried out correctly. You may feel 'worked over', but this should be an invigorating feeling and not an exhausted, painful or bruised feeling.

During detox massage is wonderful. The lighter strokes relax and warm you, the deeper strokes sort out your muscles and increase the circulation to help the internal cleansing process, and the invigorating strokes stimulate and give you a truly vital feeling. Can you tell that I trained as a massage therapist?

An Important Distinction

A common mistake to make is to think that aromatherapy and massage are the same thing. Aromatherapy massage treatments are designed to facilitate the optimum absorption of the essential oils. The treatment warms the flesh, which increases the circulation so that the body can totally absorb the oils. It is the therapeutic qualities of the oils that work and trigger effects within the body whilst the client receives the treatment, and not the physical treatment itself.

Massage treatments are designed to improve the body's circulation, lymph flow and immune system entirely through the physical use of different speed, length and pressure of strokes. You will feel much more 'worked' after a massage treatment than you should after an aromatherapy treatment.

Each of these techniques is valuable in its own right, and clients should be aware of the difference in technique in order to decide which is best for them. A sore back the day after a full afternoon of gardening can be treated by either aromatherapy or massage, but see how the approach varies. Massage would warm and stretch the muscles so that the tension is soothed and the circulation to the muscles increased to help them work efficiently. A combination of deep friction work and stretching strokes would be recommended. Aromatherapy oils such as ginger and black pepper are warming to the muscles, so would be used in combination with long, slow strokes, increasing the blood supply to the surface of the flesh to ensure the optimum absorption of oils. The results would be the same in either case – a fully relaxed body with stretched and relaxed muscles.

REFLEXOLOGY

This technique is based on the principle of reflex points or zones on the feet relating to points, organs and systems within the body. By working with these zones or points the practitioner can treat areas of illness, imbalance or weakness. It is a very old technique, recorded as far back as ancient Egyptian times. Reflexology is an excellent diagnostic tool as it can reveal any problems within the body, even at early stages. The practitioner can then work on them before any further, more serious conditions develop.

During a reflexology treatment the client sits or lies on a treatment couch whilst the practitioner follows a sequence around each foot that covers every reflex point or zone. The practitioner will ask the client to identify areas of discomfort or pain, which can then be 'worked' to improve the condition. Reflexology practitioners often use calendula powder or ordinary talc to make the treatment go smoothly.

During the Detox Programme it is likely that your internal systems and organs will be working harder or differently from the way they would normally. Reflexology can help the body detox by 'balancing' organs like the kidneys and liver, helping the intestines to carry out their cleansing function without causing any unnecessary pressure or imbalance.

Reflexology can also tell you what your body requires or simply what it is going through. If you have treatments whilst you are detoxing you will often find 'tender points' in the bladder, kidney and digestive system, all of which are working hard. The practitioner will work on these specific points to bring them to optimum condition for continued cleansing.

Reflexology treatments will also show up any potential imbalance, and the practitioner can work at a preventative level. If you are super-healthy or your detox has made your body totally balanced, these treatments are just as useful for maintenance and prevention, and in any case they always offer a relaxing, soothing, hour-long treatment.

COLONIC IRRIGATION

Although it has been around since as early as 1500 BC, colonic irrigation seems to be a relatively new and experimental therapy for most people. It consists of an internal 'bath' that helps to cleanse the colon of accumulated poisons, gases, faecal matter and mucous deposits. The practitioner gently pumps filtered water into your rectum, which will start to soften and flush away any build-up of toxins and waste.

Colonic irrigation is extremely effective during the Detox Programme. While you are on the programme you will be eliminating all sources of toxins from your diet, which means that the original toxins, once eliminated in waste matter, are not replaced. But there will still be a build-up of toxins within your body from earlier. Whilst foods such as brown rice, nuts and pulses will help to break this down, colonic irrigation will speed up the process and actively flush out the detritus.

The colonics practitioner will ask you to lie on a couch or plinth, with your lower body covered with a towel or sheet. Filtered water at a carefully regulated temperature is introduced under gentle gravitational pressure through the rectum and into the colon. The practitioner will use massage to help the water soften and cleanse the colon of faecal matter and waste, which is flushed away with the waste water. The colon is worked on in stages: each time water is pumped in and flushed out, until the whole area is complete. The practitioner will also suggest how many further treatments are required, and recommend appropriate supplements to replace natural bowel fibre and flora. The entire session will last less than an hour.

Practitioners are totally aware of the 'unusual' circumstances in which they have to place their clients, and discretion and modesty are observed throughout. The after-effects of colonic irrigation are similar to those of the entire Detox Programme: a feeling of wellbeing, lightness, mental clarity and increased energy, a loss of any bloated feeling, relief from constipation and clearer, glowing skin.

Colonics is not something that normally springs to mind as a complementary therapy – people normally think of massage or aromatherapy. But if you have ever thought about trying this treatment to see what the effects would be, or if you believe it might help but have never got round to booking a session, this is the time to try! It's painless, it's different, it makes you feel great, and it's detoxifying.

MOISTURISING

During the Detox Programme you will be doing many new and different things to your body, most of which will cause an increased level of activity either internally or externally. During any process the body will be using up fluids in exercise, sweating, cell regeneration, elimination of toxins, cleansing and so on. This fluid must be replaced if your body is to maintain optimum levels of detoxing.

You already know that you need to drink at least 3 pints (1.7 litres) of water a day to keep your fluid levels steady, but you also need to make sure that other kinds of moisture are topped up. Each time you bath, wash, receive a treatment or carry out any of the body care treatments essential to the Detox Programme, you should moisturise your skin.

Maintaining the skin moisture levels on your body as well as your face is important to detox. Keeping the cells and flesh in good condition will help to:

- give your skin a warm glow

- allow your skin to shed old dead cells more effectively

- stop your skin looking dry and dull

A daily skin care routine is essential if you want it to stay in optimum condition. Remember, it is better to do a little and often (simply wash with water and follow with a moisturiser every day), than to do a lot infrequently (cleanse, tone, scrub, face mask and exfoliate once a month or when you can remember). Despite what the ads would have us believe, creams and gels are not the only way to keep the skin's natural moisture levels – oils are just as effective, if not better.

10

The Only Way to Banish Cellulite

Cellulite is one of the most hotly debated subjects in the health and beauty world. It has been around for ever, but the recent development of many so-called anti-cellulite creams and lotions by the cosmetics industry has given us hope. For a price, we are now led to believe that we can 'reduce the effects of cellulite' or banish it altogether. The truth is that, unless we undergo surgery, the only way to get rid of cellulite or actually to improve the condition is to change what we feed our bodies, how we exercise our bodies and how we treat our bodies.

Most of us Western women have cellulite because of our lifestyle – our diet and level of activity – rather than the genes we inherit, so this is something that we *can* change if we want to. Oriental women, with a different lifestyle and different diet, are less likely to develop cellulite. That said, some cultures are less prone to it than others simply because general body proportions and fat cell distribution vary between different cultures.

Contrary to popular belief, female hormones don't actually cause cellulite, although they do assist its progress. This helps to explain why it is more likely to develop during puberty, pregnancy and the menopause –

times when hormones are disrupted. In the same way, women who take hormone supplements such as the contraceptive pill or HRT will also be altering the body's normal state and may increase bloating, or the body's ability to process fluids and lymph efficiently.

Unfortunately, however, cellulite doesn't just disappear when hormonal shifts stop. Although our bodies all have the same number of fat cells, hormones determine their size, shape, accumulation and distribution. Stress, a sedentary lifestyle, dress, posture, bad circulation, diet and bingeing all contribute to its formation.

Men also get cellulite. Their hormones programme it to collect above and around their waist, where their fat cells are more concentrated, whereas female hormones programme it to collect on the hips and thighs where fat is concentrated in readiness for childbirth. Cellulite also looks different on men because their connective tissue is firmer and more tightly packed, and because their skin is thicker and has a higher percentage of muscle fibre – 40–45 per cent compared with 30 per cent in women.

When the circulation becomes sluggish, toxins, waste products and slow-moving lymph fluid collects between these connective tissues, resulting in cellulite. Its superficial appearance can vary widely. Some people develop a fairly consistent 'orange peel' effect, whilst others have irregular lumps, and sometimes cellulite is barely noticeable because that person's skin is so well toned.

So how do we change the factors that we *can* influence? How do we stop the circulation becoming sluggish, and the lymph flow slowing down and collecting between the connective tissue? How do we get rid of all the other lifestyle factors that increase our propensity to develop cellulite? It's a question of bringing the body back into balance and maintaining this state. The answer is quite simple – detox! The Detox Programme is the only truly effective anti-cellulite programme. Diet is addressed, exercise is addressed, posture is addressed, the skin is addressed and all relevant treatments are addressed. So the good news is that if you are on the Detox Programme you will inevitably reduce or eradicate any cellulite you might have – what a side-effect!

A CLOSER LOOK AT THE CAUSES

By taking a closer look at the causes of cellulite you will see how the Detox Programme really is the only solution.

Poor eating habits

The down-side of convenience foods

If you don't watch what you eat or you eat 'on the hoof', grabbing pre-packed foods or ready-meals, it is likely that your diet will be high in fats and sugars. When these are broken down by the metabolism much of the product is surplus to nutritional requirements, and the result is fat. In women this fat naturally accumulates around the thigh and buttock area. Extra weight places a strain on the skin cells and tissue. The constant weakening of this tissue will eventually result in permanent weakness, which manifests itself in sagging, drooping flesh. This lack of skin tone is likely to make the cellulite more visible.

Diets and binges

If you continually change the way you eat, one week eating masses of food and the following week next to nothing because you are 'dieting', your body will do everything in its power to reduce this fluctuation – it goes into 'starvation mode'. To regulate the peaks and troughs of diet/binge eating, the metabolism slows down in order not to burn the fat. By doing so, it will have stores of fat to use as energy the next time it is starved. The result is that, even if you 'diet', you don't lose weight. If you start to increase the quantities you eat over a short period of time your body is not ready to deal with the overload – it is not in a position automatically to raise its metabolic rate – and so you feel bloated, your circulation and lymph system are over-stretched, and you cannot process the waste and excess efficiently. This results in the waste being stored in the body and increases the occurrence of cellulite.

The perils of an imbalanced diet

If you eat an imbalanced diet you will not be providing your body with the essential nutrients it requires to process food and maintain your body in peak condition. A diet full of ready-made, pre-packed or processed foods is a diet full of colourings, flavourings, preservatives and sweeteners. It is also probably a sodium-dominant diet (see p.184). There may not be enough fibre in the diet, and the 'fresh foods' content will be almost non-existent. When the body has been fuelled by such sub-standard nutrients over an extended period of time the result will be tiredness and lethargy, muscle aches and fatigue.

Unidentified food intolerances

Personal food intolerances, if not heeded, can result in a build-up of substances that the body finds difficult to process. Many people have an intolerance to certain foods, the most common of which are:

- All dairy products
- Caffeine
- Alcohol
- Malt
- Yeast
- Wheat-based products (flour, bread, pasta etc.)
- Barley
- Maize
- Rye
- Refined flours
- Chocolate
- Refined sugar
- Refined starch

The easy way to detect an intolerance is to identify what you depend on in your diet and what you crave. The foods which you eat a lot of and regularly, such as bread and cheese, may be doing more harm than good and should be reduced or eliminated from your diet.

The sodium/potassium imbalance

The careful balance of potassium and sodium in our bodies is crucial to the efficient flow of oxygen, essential nutrients and waste to and from our cells. Sodium is found mainly inside the cells and potassium outside the cells. Essentially the sodium/potassium balance within the body creates a fully functioning 'pump' – sodium absorbs and potassium expels. If this pump is imbalanced and the sodium is allowed to become dominant, movement between cells becomes sluggish, the removal of waste slows down and leads to build-up, fluid is retained and congestion occurs. The short-term effects are bloating and fluid retention, the long-term ones bad cell renewal and regeneration, which damages the internal structure of the cells.

All processed foods contain added salt. We typically add salt when we cook food and add more on the plate when we sit down to eat. Our taste buds are so used to salt that we gradually increase our tolerance, and in turn our intake.

It is very difficult on a day-to-day basis to include enough potassium in the diet to balance the high levels of sodium. Potassium is found in large quantities in fresh fruit, fresh vegetables, sprouted beans and sprouted seeds. Your diet needs to contain twice as much potassium as sodium in order to create a healthy flow of nutrients and efficient expulsion of waste. There are various ways in which you can do this:

- Avoid processed, canned and ready-made foods

- Never add salt when cooking and reduce the amount of

salt you put on your plate. Taste the food first and then only add salt in small amounts. We automatically add salt without giving the taste of the food a chance first

- If your food seems short on flavour look to other seasonings and herbs for an alternative: cayenne pepper, black or white pepper, garlic etc. will all add flavour and possibly introduce a new taste experience as well as extra nutrients

- Canned fish often comes in brine, which is salt water. Canned vegetables come in water with added salt. If you rinse these before eating them you will dramatically reduce your salt intake

- Beware the word 'sodium' in an ingredient – it means salt. Always read the ingredients lists on packaged foods (bicarbonate of soda = sodium bicarbonate; mono-sodium glutamate, sodium sulphite and sodium benzoate are all commonly found)

- Increase your intake of potassium-rich foods such as potatoes, melon, carrots, broccoli, papaya, watermelon, Brussels sprouts and all fresh vegetables

- Eat more beans (kidney beans, black beans, aduki beans etc.)

- Eat your vegetables raw. Alternatively, cook them in the smallest possible amount of water or steam them lightly. Better still, use the liquid you cooked the vegetables in to make soup or stock

STRESS

You may not easily make the connection between stress and cellulite, and it is even more unlikely that you will make the connection between stress and the sodium/potassium balance in the body. But there most certainly is a connection, and it goes like this. Stressful situations trigger a release of the hormone adrenaline to various relevant parts of the body – legs to run away, to the shoulders and arms to fight etc. This is the fight-or-flight response that was explained earlier. Adrenaline is used for many other functions including water regulation. Increased stress levels cause increased release of adrenaline, which causes imbalance in potassium/sodium levels, which causes bloating and fluid retention.

Stress is also a self-perpetuating condition. We are stressed and we get tired. We do not or cannot do anything about reducing the stress. This becomes stressful in itself and we become even more stressed (and so on and so on).

If you are under stress you should try to look at the causes and then make some changes to your life that will alleviate or remove the triggers. In the meantime you can introduce into your life some simple tools that will have many benefits:

- Drinking water

- Balanced, healthy diet

- Breathing techniques

- Relaxation technique

- Exercise
- Affirmations
- Positive thinking
- Massage
- Aromatherapy
- Relaxation
- Walking

All these subjects are covered in depth in chapters 4 and 9.

POSTURE AND CLOTHING

The importance of good posture

The body is designed with sufficient spacing for our internal organs and systems to function correctly and without hindrance. Changing this spacing through bad posture means the body has to operate in an unnatural and forced environment. Restricted blood flow, inability to breathe deeply, squashed flesh, restricted stomach movement and muscle shortening causes inefficient flow of blood, lymph and waste within the body. The result is congestion, which leads to cellulite.

Avoid restrictive clothing

Another way in which we destroy this spacing is by wearing restrictive clothing. Remember the fashion for purchasing a tight pair of jeans and then wearing them in the bath to shrink them even further, until the only way to get them done up was to use a hook to pull up the zip whilst wriggling on the floor? Remember the wide belts that pulled in your waist until breathing became an optional extra? Remember teetering on four-inch heels as an adolescent to try and gain those all-important inches? All these 'fashions' (and every generation has its equivalents) restrict not only normal day-to-day physical movement but also natural movement within the body. This restriction results in congestion and so increases the likelihood of cellulite.

INACTIVITY

In any one day we typically spend eight hours lying down and eight hours sitting down. The remainder is split between standing and walking. We lie down to sleep, we sit in a car, we sit on the bus, we sit on the train, we sit at a desk, we sit watching a movie, we sit watching television, we sit down to eat, we stand talking to colleagues or neighbours, we sit with young children while they are going to sleep, we sit down to rest.

We know that mobility is important in old or ill people in order to prevent muscle wastage, bed sores, weakness, oedema, bad circulation and poor respiration, but we never stop to think that any of those effects might happen to us. If it did it would be an extreme case, but if we don't take care our ankles can become bloated or our circulation sluggish just through our normal modus operandi.

Make a note of your daily activity levels. How much do

you sit down? How often do you take the car when you could walk? How often does your leisure activity include sitting or standing still? Change just one of these each day and you will notice the effects on your circulation almost immediately. Good circulation means efficient processing and elimination of waste products which in turn eliminates cellulite. Try:

- Stretching

- Exercise

- Movement of all kinds

- Cold water splashing

- Cold showers

- Saunas

Make sure you get some exercise every day. It will increase your muscle tone, which will improve the appearance of your flesh; it also increases circulation and lymph flow. Dry skin brushing (see p.59) is an excellent means of 'kick starting' the circulation first thing in the morning and last thing at night. The muscle action required to skin brush is quite vigorous in itself, but the main benefits are found in the sloughing off of dead cells, which allows the skin to breathe more efficiently, and the boost to circulation from the brushing itself. Anything you can do to extend and contract the muscles in your body will help keep your cirulation, skin tone and condition in tip-top order.

ANTI-CELLULITE CHECKLIST

The checklist below will ensure that you follow an anti-cellulite programme. All the areas are covered in depth elsewhere in the book, but this list will act as an aide-memoire towards your cellulite-free future.

- Eat fresh fruit every day

- Eat fresh vegetables every day

- Eat rice, beans and pulses every day

- Eat oily fish every day

- Where possible buy organic foods

- If you change from a diet heavy in processed foods, invest in a good vitamin supplement – multivitamins with no added yeast, flour or talcum

- Avoid drugs, prescribed or other

- Avoid hormone pills

- Eliminate processed foods

- Eliminate pre-packed foods

- Eliminate ready-made meals

- Drink at least 3 pints (1.7 litres) of water a day

- Drink herbal teas or hot water with lemon and honey

- Limit your dairy foods or eliminate them altogether

- Reduce your fat intake

- Reduce your sugar intake
- Reduce your salt intake
- Do more exercise
- Adjust your posture – don't cross your legs!
- Reduce any stress in your life and avoid stressful situations
- Dry skin brush every morning
- Dry skin brush every evening
- Self massage every morning
- Self massage every evening
- Cold shower or cold bath every day
- Moisturise your skin every day
- Breathe deeply
- Smile

Useful Addresses

Contact the appropriate organisation for names of fully qualified, registered practitioners in your local area. The first two organisations are concerned with all forms of therapy, including massage; the others are self-explanatory.

British Complementary Medicine Association
9 Soar Lane
Leicester
LE3 5DE
tel. 0116 242 5406

Institute for Complementary Medicine
PO Box 194
London SE16 1QZ
tel. 0171 237 5165

Aromatherapy Organisations Council
3 Latymer Close
Braybrooke
Market Harborough
LE16 8LN
tel. 01858 434242

Colonic International Association
16 Englands Lane
London NW3 4TG
tel. 0171 483 1595

Association of Reflexologists
27 Old Gloucester Street
London WC1 3XX
tel. 0990 673320

Index

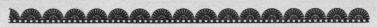

THE BRITISH SCHOOL OF COMPLEMENTARY THERAPY
140 Harley Street, London W1N 1AH

On production of this coupon you are entitled to **10% off** any course or treatment you book in either London or Stratford-upon-Avon. Massage, aromatherapy and reflexology treatments are available to combine with your Detox Programme.

Brochures giving details of treatments, courses and dates are available. Please write to the above address, enclosing an A5 stamped, addressed envelope.

Keep this coupon until any payment is required – and reduction will be made at time of purchase. Do not send the coupon with your brochure request.

Please send a copy of your brochure to:

NAME _____

ADDRESS _____

_____

_____

TELEPHONE No. (HOME) _____

(WORK) _____

Send to: The BSCT, 140 Harley Street, London W1N 1AH